the Pilates Program *for* Every Body

CAROLAN BROWN

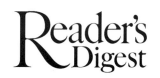

Reader's Digest

A READER'S DIGEST BOOK
Published by The Reader's Digest Association in arrangement with Tucker Slingsby Ltd.

Library of Congress Cataloging-in-Publication Data

Brown, Carolan.
   The pilates program for every body : easy routines for every
age / Carolan Brown.
      p.cm.
   Includes index.
   ISBN 13: 978-0-7621-0451-2
   ISBN 10: 0-7621-0451-1
   1. Pilates method. I. Title.

RA781.B757 2004
613.7'1–dc21

                        2003047227

FOR TUCKER SLINGSBY
Editorial: Sally Harding, Del Tucker
Design: Helen Mathias, Robert Mathias, Steve Rowling
Illustrations: Robert Mathias
Photography: Andrew Sydenham
Index: Mary Warren
Models' outfits from WORKOUT— www.workoutweybridge.co.uk

FOR READER'S DIGEST
U.S. Project Editor: Miranda Smith
Canadian Project Editor: Pamela Johnson
Project Designer: George McKeon
Executive Editor, Trade Publishing: Dolores York
Senior Design Director: Michele Laseau
Director, Trade Publishing: Christopher T. Reggio
Vice President & Publisher, Trade Publishing: Harold Clarke

A NOTE TO OUR READERS

It is always advisable to check with your doctor before starting any exercise program. Consult your doctor about any symptoms that may require diagnosis or medical attention. Pregnant women are particularly advised to consult their doctor before starting Pilates practice. While the advice and information in this book is believed to be accurate and the exercises have been devised to avoid strain, neither the author, the publisher, nor the copyright holder can accept any legal responsibility for any injury sustained while doing the poses and exercises in this book.

Address any comments about *The Pilates Program for Every Body* to:
The Reader's Digest Association, Inc., Adult Trade Publishing, Reader's Digest Road, Pleasantville, NY 10570-7000

For Reader's Digest products and information, visit our website:
www.rd.com (in the United States)   www.readersdigest.ca (in Canada)

Manufactured in China
9 10 8

Contents

Pilates is for everybody

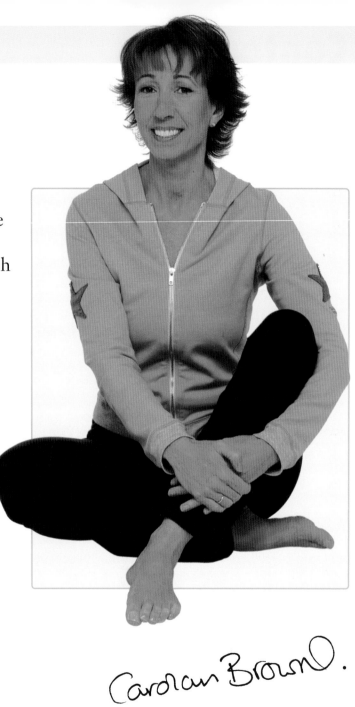

Pilates is no longer the world's best-kept secret for keeping strong and supple. The secret's out and now everyone can benefit from the simple but powerful exercises devised by Joseph Pilates. The Pilates method was originally used by dancers, athletes, and performers to help them maintain lithe, lean, and mobile bodies. It has now evolved to suit everybody's needs and has become a tried and tested program based on long-term, consistent results.

Joseph Pilates realized how much our lifestyles affect the way our bodies work. For many of us today, periods of sitting too long at a desk or in the car lead to poor posture and weak muscles. The Pilates method is a sensible and effective way to keep your body in shape however busy and stressed your lifestyle. It treats your body as a whole—lengthening and strengthening muscles and training your mind to control the way you move.

My step-by-step guide to the Pilates method will introduce you to the unique exercises that I have created following the "fit to function" philosophy of Joseph Pilates. I have been teaching this program to my students for the last 20 years. High repetitions are not part of Pilates. By using your mind to control the way you exercise, you need only do 5 or 6 repetitions. This makes my program an exercise regime that will fit into your busy schedule.

You will discover the basics of good posture, powerful breathing techniques, and the fundamental exercises that will lengthen and strengthen your muscles. This is a complete exercise program that will make you look and feel great. I hope you will get hooked on Pilates as I did and will make my program as much a part of your daily routine as brushing your teeth. It is well worth it!

Carolan Brown.

1 About Pilates

The story of Pilates

"A man is as old as his spine is flexible!"—Joseph Pilates 1880–1967

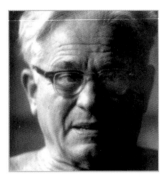

Joseph Pilates (pronounced pi-LAH-teez), the founder of the Pilates method of exercise, was still training athletes, dancers, celebrities, and businessmen until he was well into his 80s. But as a child, Pilates was frail and weak. It was to strengthen his own body that compelled him to develop his unique fitness regime.

Later in life he explained, "I picked up my knowledge as a child watching men at work and at play. Then I watched animals [in the zoo]...and discovered that [they] had the best method of keeping fit. With just a little daily stretching and balancing on the edge of rocks or on branches of trees in their cage, [big cats] can keep themselves fit." To exercises based on these observations, he added what he judged to be the most effective elements from many disciplines including gymnastics, skiing, diving, yoga, and dance. "You don't need weights or machinery to keep you fit," he said, "you just need regular functional exercise like stretching and flexing muscles, balancing, and using your own body weight as resistance."

The Pilates technique develops

Pilates was born in Germany. As a young man he overcame the physical problems of his childhood to work as a tumbler in the circus. When the First World War broke out in 1914, Pilates found himself working in England and, along with many other Germans, was interned in a prisoner of war camp on the Isle of Man. During his stay there, he helped many of the internees stay physically fit with his training programs. After the war, Pilates first returned to Germany where he trained military police in physical fitness. Then he decided to travel overseas. He arrived in the United States in 1925 and, using his formulated series of exercises, then called Contrology, he set up his first studio. His exercises became increasingly popular with dancers who found the Pilates method ideal for maintaining healthy performing bodies.

Joseph Pilates's training method has been preserved, passed on, and refined over the past 80 years. It was, until recently, perhaps the world's best-kept secret for getting and keeping strong and supple. Now the Pilates program is popular worldwide and people everywhere are enjoying its benefits.

A unique form of simple, precise, and effective exercise, Pilates is gentle on the body but offers amazing benefits—focusing as it does on the deep muscles responsible for your body's core strength and stability. It has become known as the thinking person's workout. The exercises require a mental focus that helps you to develop a greater understanding of how your body works. When you understand how your body works, you can make it work more efficiently.

Pilates exercises strengthen the joints and muscles used in everyday actions like walking, sitting, twisting, bending, and lifting—unlike traditional fitness training, which often bears little relation to our everyday movements. In time, with Pilates training, the "correct" movements become automatic and you will sit, stand, and move well all through your day.

Good posture, good health

The main aim of Pilates is to improve your posture by strengthening the stabilizing muscles of the torso. Though good posture may sound like a modest aim, your posture has a profound effect on your general physical fitness and well-being. Imbalances in the spine can cause serious injury and lead to early aging (see page 8).

Exercises for every body

It takes a little time—and regular exercise—to understand and learn the principles of the Pilates technique. Start by leaving your preconceptions behind and be patient. Take time to understand the new principles and allow your mind and body to adjust. The beauty of the exercises chosen for this book is that they are suitable for all levels of fitness and for all ages and can even be done safely by those who have experienced back pain or injury to their spine.

Pilates plus points

- Better posture and improved coordination
- Ability to move well and freely
- Good mental focus
- Automatic use of correct, efficient body movements—prevents strains and pains
- Increased muscular strength and flexibility
- Good fitness level and muscle tone
- Firm, flattened abdominal muscles
- A body that looks and feels younger

Before there were time- and labor-saving gadgets like computers and washing machines, cars for transport, and televisions for entertainment, we were all more active and our bodies had to work much harder.

Today, most of us have sedentary jobs and hectic lifestyles. We live with increasing amounts of stress and long workdays, often bringing up a family and holding down a full-time job. Excessive amounts of stress, combined with long periods of physical inactivity, can have a very bad effect on your health and well-being.

Signs of stress

Many people enjoy working under stress and thrive on the adrenaline rush. In a perfect world the stress of new challenges is beneficial and makes you feel alive and stimulated.

However, if too many stress factors come along at once, it's easy to suffer from overload. The result can be a negative outlook, lack of energy, and constant tiredness that can lead to illness and depression.

Lack of correct exercise

A sedentary lifestyle can result in muscles that are weak. Weak muscles can lead to poor posture, ill health, organ-related diseases such as heart disease, and respiratory problems. Effects that are all too often put down to the results of

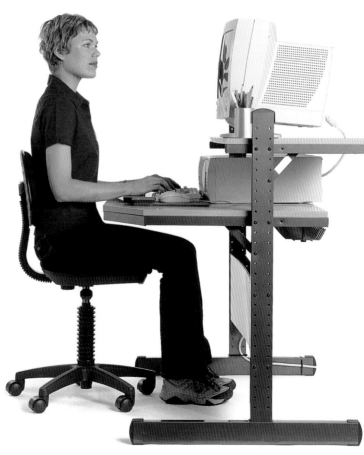

increasing age but are actually avoidable.

Always being in a rush does not mean you have exercised! In fact, it can mean the opposite. All you have done is increase your stress levels, which can lead to tight, aching muscles, and untold strain on the internal organs that are often recruited into this frenzied activity.

Pilates—a life-changing technique

Pilates fits with a busy lifestyle. It doesn't require expensive equipment or lots of space, and you can practice at home. Movements are slow and controlled. This minimizes the possibility of injury, so just about anybody of any age or fitness level can learn it.

The deep breathing that is part of the program helps to reduce stress and calm your mind and body. The improved core stability you will gain from the exercises helps you maintain a good posture, improved balance, and more coordinated, youthful movements.

Pilates looks after your posture and helps you maintain the strong, flexible spine you need to stand, sit, and move well. Good posture makes you stronger and more confident, with a greater range of movement. Combined with the toned muscles that Pilates also gives you, good posture makes you look longer, leaner, and years younger! A strong spine will also prevent injury as well as aches and pains from daily activities. If you are keen on sports or a regular exerciser, good posture will improve your performance and breathing, too.

Body awareness

Our bodies are so good at adapting to our lifestyles that we do not always realize that we are developing postural problems until we experience pain. Pilates helps by teaching you how to be aware of your posture as you move and sit every day—and how to improve it. By encouraging you to focus your mind on your body when exercising, Pilates gives you a better understanding of how your body works—alerting you to imbalances or weaknesses.

Functioning well

Pilates exercises your abdominal muscles correctly and efficiently, so you will gain good core stability and good posture faster than with more traditional fitness methods.

Many fashionable training methods involve lifting heavy weights and working isolated muscle groups in a single direction or plane of motion. They work on the muscles nearest the surface of your body, leaving the important, deeper muscles weaker. The results of lifting weights might be good for your image in a bikini or shorts, but this form of exercise can create an imbalance in your body.

In Pilates, you will work the abdominal muscles in many different planes—standing, sitting, on all fours, lying face down, on your side, and on your back. In this way you will learn how to engage your muscles to maintain balance and core stability.

Your spine

As the central structure of your skeleton, your spine gets the most attention during Pilates exercises. The spine is made up of a series of joints, called vertebrae. The discs between the vertebrae act as shock absorbers, cushioning the vertebrae as they move.

The spine has four natural curves. These curves help the body remain in balance, bear weight, absorb shocks, and flex and extend.

The spine (side view)

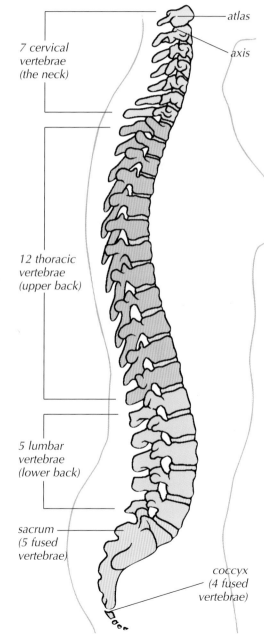

atlas

axis

7 cervical vertebrae (the neck)

12 thoracic vertebrae (upper back)

5 lumbar vertebrae (lower back)

sacrum (5 fused vertebrae)

coccyx (4 fused vertebrae)

Each bone in your body is linked to the next by ligaments and tendons forming a joint. Each joint has its own degree of mobility. Keeping the muscles around your joints strong and flexible keeps your joints mobile and helps prevent youthful flexibility from deteriorating into the stiffness of old age.

Pilates focuses on the main joints of the body that are essential for good movement, balance, and posture. These are the spine, the shoulder girdle, and the pelvic girdle.

The spine is divided into vertebrae, most of which are jointed and flexible. The skull pivots on the first vertebra called the atlas. The atlas bone can rock backward and forward, allowing the head to nod; the second vertebra, called the axis, allows the head to move from side to side.

The shoulder girdle is made up of the shoulder blades and the collarbones. Weak or unbalanced muscles holding these joints can result in round shoulders and restricted movement. The pelvic girdle is the largest and heaviest bone in your body. Its correct alignment is vital to good posture.

Lordosis and kyphosis

The most common spinal conditions are lordosis and kyphosis. The hollow in the lower back is called the lumbar curve, or lordosis, and the depth of the natural curve varies from person to person. This curve is lost when you round your back by bending forward or when you are slouching in a chair. If the lordosis is lost often and for long periods, back problems can occur.

Kyphosis is an over-curvature of the thoracic spine that creates round shoulders and a hump back. It often affects the neck, making the chin poke forward. Sufferers often have tight neck and chest muscles which can restrict circulation around vital organs and affect general health.

Bones and joints of the torso

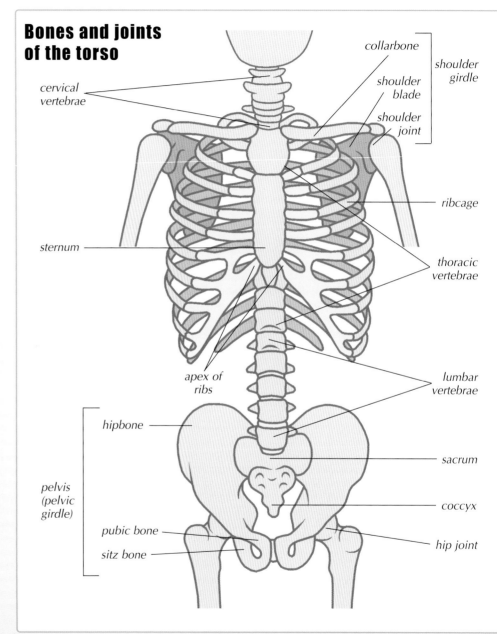

collarbone

shoulder girdle

cervical vertebrae

shoulder blade

shoulder joint

ribcage

sternum

thoracic vertebrae

apex of ribs

lumbar vertebrae

hipbone

sacrum

pelvis (pelvic girdle)

coccyx

pubic bone

hip joint

sitz bone

Pectoral muscles

Latissimus dorsi

Erector muscles

BACK

Rectus abdominus

External obliques

ABDOMEN

Internal obliques

Quadratus lumborum

Gluteus maximus (buttocks)

Pelvic floor muscles

Hip flexor and quadriceps muscles

Intercostal muscles (between ribs)

Hamstrings

Movement is created when one muscle contracts and another releases. Muscles work in opposing pairs—when one muscle contracts, the opposing muscle relaxes, allowing the movement to take place.

The main muscles responsible for good posture are the core stabilizing muscles—abdominal, back, and pelvic floor muscles. They are attached to the spine. Joseph Pilates called these muscles the "powerhouse." When they are strong, these muscles stabilize the torso in a good posture that allows the limbs to move freely without strain.

The muscles we concentrate on in Pilates exercises are shown here. Called the "girdle of steel" because it wraps around the body from back to front, the transversus muscle is the key muscle of the powerhouse.

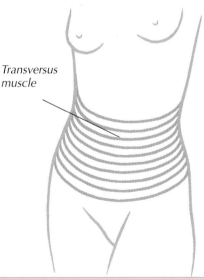

The girdle of steel

Transversus muscle

This book is divided into three main sections. Chapters 1, 2, and 3 look at the basics of Pilates.

Chapter 1 explains the principles of Pilates exercises and which muscles and bones affect posture and mobility.

Chapters 2 and 3 show you how to align your body correctly, and how to breathe deeply while keeping your body correctly aligned.

The workouts

The exercises in Chapters 4 to 9 form the basis of all your Pilates workouts. Each chapter is based on standing, lying, kneeling, or sitting and each features a range of exercises photographed step by step so you can follow exactly what to do. There are also suggestions for adapting poses to suit your level of flexibility. Each chapter ends with a short workout that will encourage you to practice the new exercises. Work through the chapters in order, moving on to each new chapter when you feel confident with the last.

The Fast-Track Workout (Chapter 10) pulls together the exercises you have learned from previous chapters into one flowing exercise routine. This workout takes 15–20 minutes and will leave you feeling stretched, energized, and alive! Practice it regularly—ideally around two or three times a week—and you will achieve a flatter stomach; a better aligned, more elegant posture; and increased strength and flexibility. In time, your body will look longer and leaner.

Taking it further

Chapter 11 shows you how to fit more challenging exercises into your regular workout as your strength and flexibility increase. And Chapter 12 gives specially selected Pilates exercises that are helpful if you have back problems or tense, over-tight muscles.

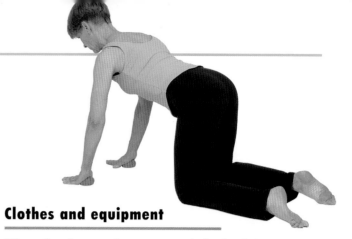

Clothes and equipment

You don't need any special clothing or equipment. Simply choose clothes that allow you to move freely. Practice in a room with enough space to be able to stretch out to the sides and above your head, both when standing and lying on the floor. An exercise mat with a nonslip surface is useful to protect you from a cold, hard floor and help your feet and hands stay in position. A cushion and towel may also be helpful for some exercises and details are given throughout the book where appropriate.

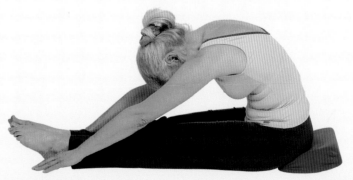

CHAPTER 2

Neutral Spine

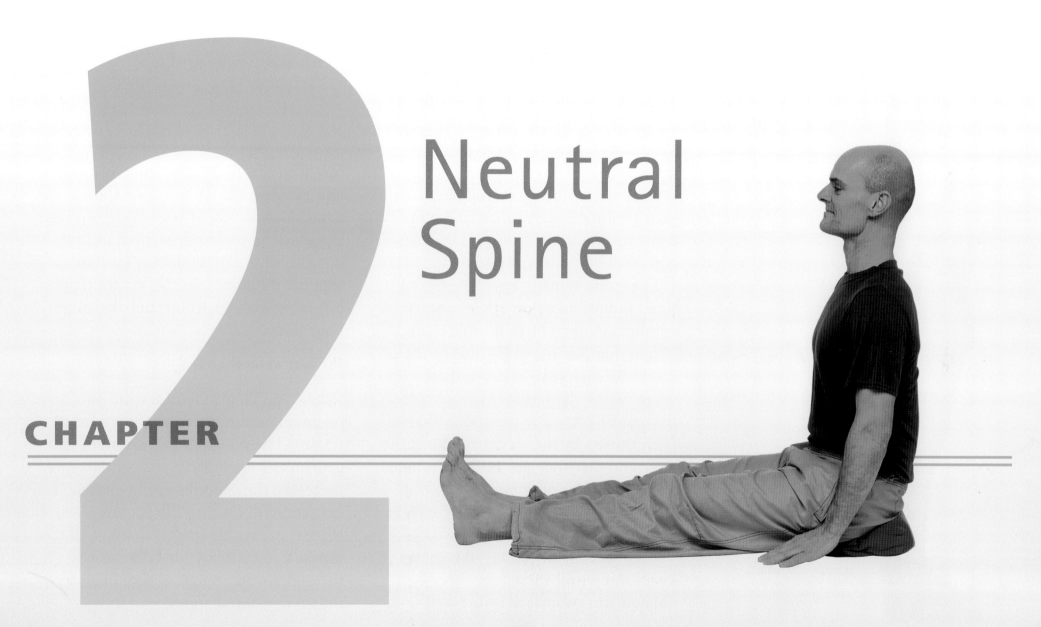

About neutral spine

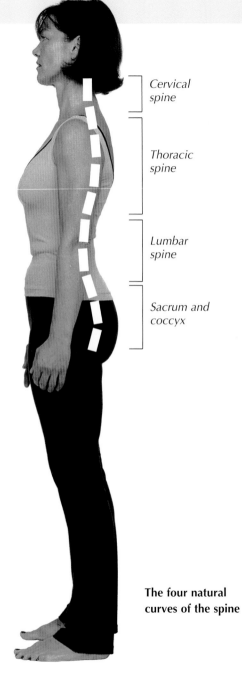

Cervical spine

Thoracic spine

Lumbar spine

Sacrum and coccyx

The four natural curves of the spine

People come in lots of different shapes and sizes, but the basic design of the skeleton is the same for everyone and its alignment is the key to good posture.

The spine is the central axis of the skeleton. When it is well aligned and your posture is well balanced, you put less stress on your joints and muscles as you go about your daily activities.

The spine is made up of a series of small bones linked together by muscles and ligaments to form flexible joints. When muscles are weak or tight they can unbalance your body, pulling your spine out of alignment. Most people have some muscular imbalance that has been caused by the way they move, the wear and tear they put on their joints, or by lack of regular exercise.

What is neutral spine?

When your major joints—the ankles, knees, hips, and shoulders—are aligned and your back is in a well-balanced position, your spine is in its neutral position. When your spine is in neutral, each side of your body carries an equal amount of body weight and the muscles of the body do not have to support the joints. In this position you can move easily without unbalancing your body.

The four natural curves

When you view a neutral spine in profile, you can see it has four natural curves. These curves give strength and protect the spine from impact damage; therefore they should not be flattened or exaggerated. During Pilates exercises, the natural curves are retained at all times. Even when your body moves through a wide range, it should always return to neutral spine.

For most people, backache and other postural problems stem from the way they move. How we sit and stand, as well as lift and carry heavy items affects body alignment, as do postural changes that occur during pregnancy and labor. Even the way we move while overcoming an injury can have long-term effects on our posture.

The keys to a well-aligned and well-balanced posture are to remain supple and maintain good joint mobility, good pelvic and shoulder alignment, and strong, lengthened muscles. Gentle, flowing Pilates exercises focus on all these elements.

Pelvic alignment is essential for good posture. The pelvis is the largest bone in the body and is attached to the largest muscles in the body. It is the base from which the rest of your body extends. Correct alignment and movement of the pelvis prevents lower-back pain and helps to maintain a healthy spine. The ability to control the alignment of your pelvis by using your abdominal muscles while your limbs are moving is the focus of many Pilates exercises. Gaining this ability gives strength and stability to your body.

Many people carry tension in the neck and shoulder area and this tension can have an effect on your shoulder alignment. Learning to relax the shoulders and strengthen the neck and shoulder girdle helps improve the range of movement in the upper body and release unnecessary tension.

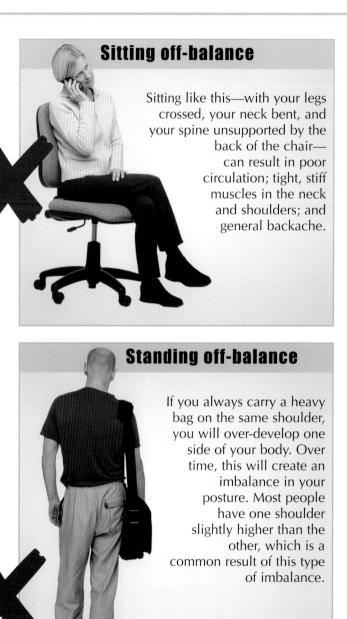

Sitting off-balance

Sitting like this—with your legs crossed, your neck bent, and your spine unsupported by the back of the chair—can result in poor circulation; tight, stiff muscles in the neck and shoulders; and general backache.

Well-aligned sitting

To support your spine, sit back in the chair. Keep your legs uncrossed and your feet on the floor. Make sure your shoulders are directly above your hips and keep your head well aligned and your neck lengthened. Place a cushion behind the lumbar area of your back if you need more support.

Standing off-balance

If you always carry a heavy bag on the same shoulder, you will over-develop one side of your body. Over time, this will create an imbalance in your posture. Most people have one shoulder slightly higher than the other, which is a common result of this type of imbalance.

Well-aligned standing

The correct way to carry a shoulder bag is to place the strap over the shoulder opposite the weight of the bag. If your bag does not have a shoulder strap, frequently change sides. However, the best option is not to carry a heavy bag unless it is absolutely necessary!

Before trying Pilates exercises you need to learn how to move your spine into its neutral position. Start moving your spine into alignment from the feet up. Breathe deeply a few times to relax, then follow the exercise below to position your feet, moving gently and slowly. Correct foot placement allows you to start aligning the joints, beginning with ankles, knees, and hips. Make sure that your feet do not roll outward or inward and that your weight is evenly distributed between the balls and the heels of the feet. Check that your knees are not rolling inward and are very slightly bent—this is

called having soft knee joints. You will be less likely to injure your joints if you learn to stand with soft knee joints rather than locked ones.

If you have bad postural habits, you may feel awkward and off-balance when you first move your feet into the correct position. To regain a comfortable balance, practice the foot placement exercises shown to the right. You will gradually feel rooted and stable in your standing position and ready to progress to the next stage of getting into neutral spine—aligning your pelvis.

Foot placement exercises

With your feet parallel, roll them inward and outward a few times, then find the correct position with the weight evenly balanced.

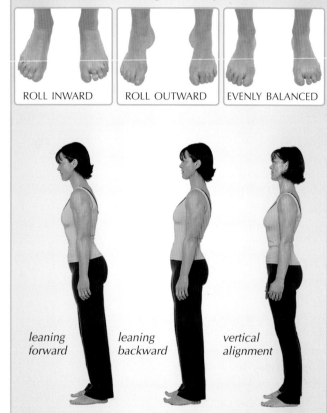

ROLL INWARD | ROLL OUTWARD | EVENLY BALANCED

leaning forward | *leaning backward* | *vertical alignment*

Rock forward and backward on your feet to find the central position where your weight is evenly distributed between the balls and heels.

You should now have your feet in the correct position, firmly balanced and centered, with your ankles, knees, and hips in alignment.

Positioning your feet

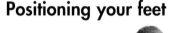

1 Stand erect with your feet together.

2 Turn your toes outward, keeping your legs and heels together.

3 Line up your heels with your toes so that your ankles, knees, and hips are in alignment. Do not lock your knees backward.

To stand in neutral spine, it is essential for your pelvis to be correctly aligned. Misalignment can often result in lower-back pain and hip problems.

To line up your pelvis, first stand with your feet in alignment (see previous page). Concentrate on extending your tailbone toward the floor, keeping your buttocks relaxed.

Your pubic bone and hipbones should be in alignment with each other. Place your fingertips over your pubic bone and the heels of your hands over your hipbones, making a V-shape. Your palms should form a level triangle perpendicular to the floor. If they aren't or you are unsure, try the exercise for aligning your pelvis.

How to check pelvic alignment

How to align your pelvis

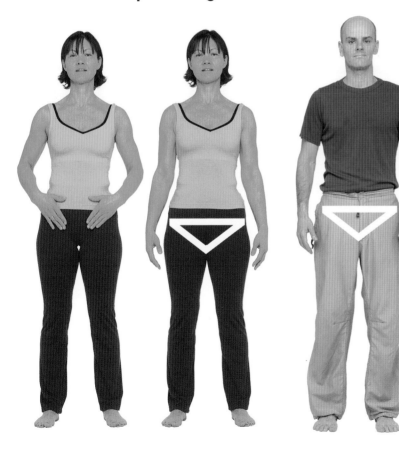

1 Stand with your feet hip-distance apart and your weight distributed evenly on each foot. Place your fingertips over your pubic bone and the heels of your hands over your hipbones, making a V-shape. Bend your knees slightly and tilt your pelvis as far forward as you can.

2 Keeping your hands where they are, tilt your pelvis as far back as you can.

3 Find the midway position between the forward and backward tilt and stand up straight. Your hands should now form a level triangle perpendicular to the floor. Your pelvis is now in neutral.

Once your weight is evenly balanced over each foot and your pelvis is in neutral, you are ready to concentrate on moving your upper body into neutral. To do this, first think about the natural curves of the spine. Above the pelvis is the lumbar curve, which should remain curved. Above the lumbar curve is the thoracic spine, which is linked to the back of the ribcage and also has a natural curve. Next, consider your ribcage area—it is a cylinder containing the vital organs. It should be in an open and lengthened position so your organs aren't compressed. To help lengthen your torso, try to imagine one piece of string attached to your breastbone and another to the middle of the back of your ribcage and that both strings are being gently pulled upward.

The shoulder girdle sits on top of your ribcage. To align this with the rest of the body, relax your shoulders back and down so that the shoulder joints are directly above the hips, knees, and ankles.

At the very top of your spine is the cervical area, or neck. Once your feet and pelvis are in alignment and you have checked the alignment of your spine, make sure your head and neck are aligned and relaxed, too. The head should be directly above the shoulders. To achieve this, pull your chin back toward your neck without dropping your forward gaze and follow the neck alignment exercise.

Standing, lying, kneeling, and sitting in neutral spine

The following six pages explain in detail how to find the correct neutral spine position when standing, lying, kneeling on all fours, and sitting. In Pilates, every exercise starts from one of these neutral spine positions.

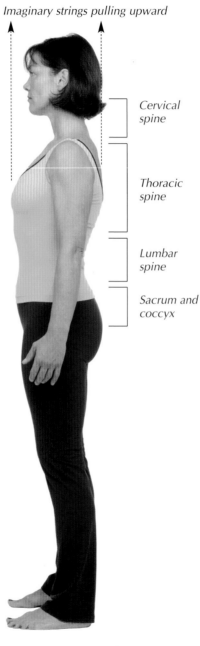

Imaginary strings pulling upward

Cervical spine

Thoracic spine

Lumbar spine

Sacrum and coccyx

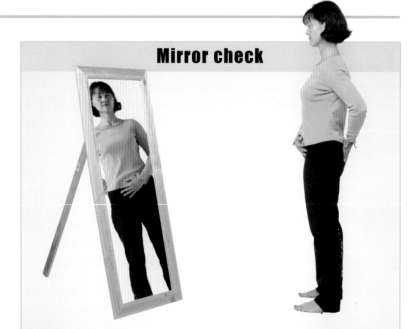

Mirror check

When you stand in neutral, you should feel stable and balanced. To study your posture, stand in front of a full-length mirror. Check that your ankles, knees, and hips are in alignment and your pelvis is in neutral, with your tailbone extending toward the floor. Your chest should be lifting upward and your shoulders should be back and down.

Aligning your neck

1. Standing in your neutral spine position, jut your chin forward.

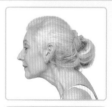

2. Draw your chin in so that your neck is lengthening and you feel that you are lifting from the top of your head. Your neck should now be in alignment.

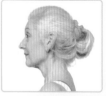

STANDING IN NEUTRAL

This page reviews all you need to do to move your spine into neutral when standing. Practice this each time you start Pilates exercises and it will soon become second nature.

Stand with your feet together. Keeping your heels and legs together, turn your toes outward. Line up your heels with your toes so that your ankles, knees, and hips are in alignment. Make sure that your feet do not roll outward or inward and that your body weight is evenly distributed between the ball and heel of each foot. Your knees should be soft (slightly bent), facing front, and not rolling inward.

Line up your pelvis by placing your fingertips over your pubic bone and the heels of your hands over the hipbones, making a V-shape. Your hands should form a level triangle perpendicular to the floor. Extend your tailbone toward the floor. Keep your buttocks relaxed.

To align the upper spine, first make sure that your lumbar curve remains concave. Lift your breastbone toward the ceiling and let your shoulders relax. To help lengthen the torso, imagine that a piece of string attached to the breastbone is being gently pulled upward.

The shoulder girdle on top of the ribcage should be relaxed back and down so that your shoulder joints are in alignment with the hips, knees, and ankles. The ribcage area, which is a cylinder containing the vital organs, should remain in an open and lengthened position so your organs aren't compressed.

Align your head over your shoulders by pulling your chin back toward your neck without dropping your chin. Feel that you are lifting from the top of your head.

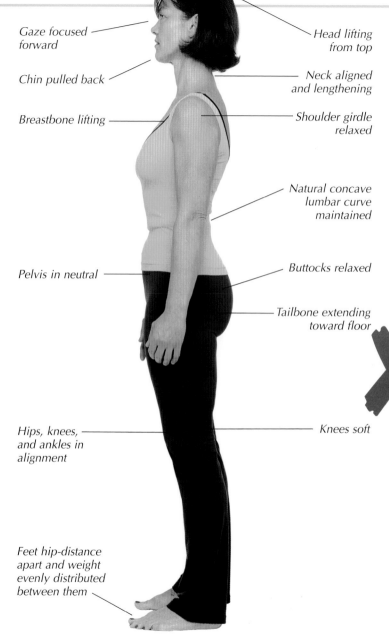

Gaze focused forward

Chin pulled back

Breastbone lifting

Pelvis in neutral

Hips, knees, and ankles in alignment

Feet hip-distance apart and weight evenly distributed between them

Head lifting from top

Neck aligned and lengthening

Shoulder girdle relaxed

Natural concave lumbar curve maintained

Buttocks relaxed

Tailbone extending toward floor

Knees soft

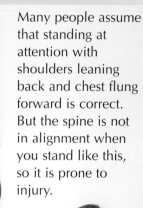

Common mistakes

Many people assume that standing at attention with shoulders leaning back and chest flung forward is correct. But the spine is not in alignment when you stand like this, so it is prone to injury.

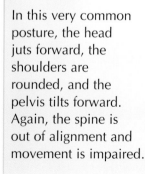

In this very common posture, the head juts forward, the shoulders are rounded, and the pelvis tilts forward. Again, the spine is out of alignment and movement is impaired.

LYING ON YOUR BACK IN NEUTRAL

Having practiced standing in neutral, you will have become more aware of the alignment of your joints and the natural curves of your spine. When practicing Pilates exercises lying on your back, you will need to start from a correct, aligned, neutral position. Only then will your body be able to flow smoothly into the various movements that will strengthen your muscles and improve your posture.

To find neutral, lie on your back with your feet flat on the floor and your knees bent and hip-distance apart. Make sure that your ankles, knees, and hips are in alignment, your feet are not rolling out, and your knees are not moving inward or outward.

Your tailbone should extend along the floor and your sacrum, the five fused vertebrae just above the tailbone, should be imprinting into the floor to place your pelvis in neutral. The thoracic spine, back of the ribs, and shoulder blades should also be imprinting into the floor. When your sacrum, shoulder blades, and upper back are imprinting into the floor, your lumbar spine should naturally curve off the floor.

Resting your head on the floor, lengthen the muscles at the back of your neck. Extend the top of your head along the floor. Make sure your chin is pulled in to help the neck muscles lengthen.

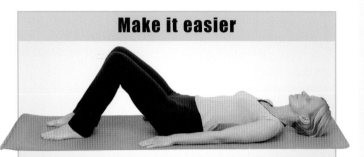

Make it easier

Lie on a mat to relieve pressure on bony joints or if the floor you are lying on is hard or cold.

Imprinting

When you imprint your bones into the mat (or the floor) you can feel them pressing down (or imprinting) into the surface below you. This will help you be aware of being in correct alignment. For example, when sitting in neutral you should feel your sitz bones pressing down into the mat (see page 24), and be aware of a slight tension in the muscles around the bones that are imprinting. In this way you will feel a connection between the joint and muscle movement.

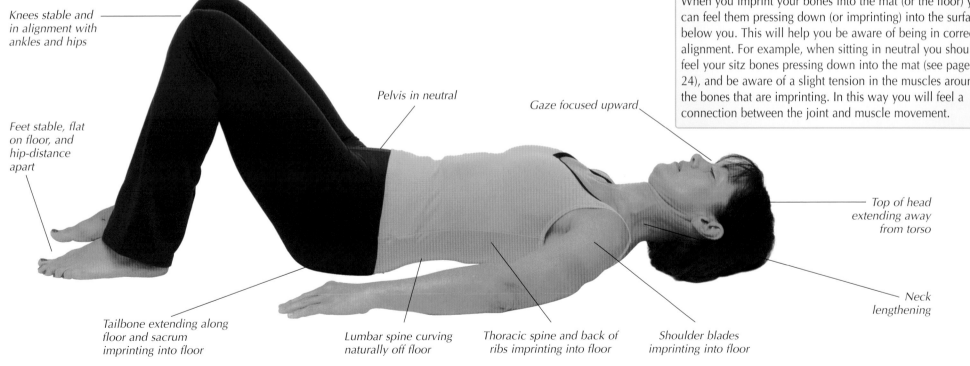

Knees stable and in alignment with ankles and hips

Feet stable, flat on floor, and hip-distance apart

Pelvis in neutral

Gaze focused upward

Top of head extending away from torso

Neck lengthening

Tailbone extending along floor and sacrum imprinting into floor

Lumbar spine curving naturally off floor

Thoracic spine and back of ribs imprinting into floor

Shoulder blades imprinting into floor

LYING ON YOUR FRONT IN NEUTRAL

For Pilates exercises practiced lying on your front, first lie face down, resting your forehead on the back of your hands. Lengthen your neck muscles by drawing your chin in and extending the top of your head away from your torso. Focus your gaze toward the floor. Draw your shoulder blades away from your neck. Completely relax the back of the ribcage and shoulder girdle.

Make sure your pubic bone and hipbones are in alignment and imprinting into the floor. Engage your pelvic floor and abdominal muscles to prevent your torso from sagging and your lumbar spine from hyperextending (over-exaggerating the lumbar curve). Extend your tailbone away from your torso. Lengthen through the legs, keeping the ankles, knees, and hips in alignment.

Engaging your muscles

To create a strong center and hold your torso in neutral, you need to engage the pelvic floor and abdominal muscles. To do this, draw up the muscles of the pelvic floor and hollow the abdominal muscles back toward the spine as you exhale. It is important not to overtighten or clench your muscles.

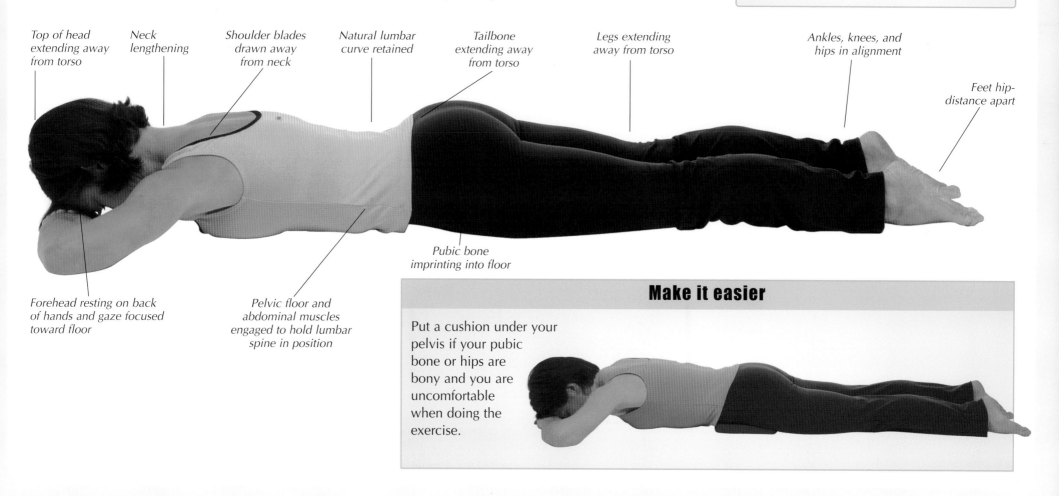

Top of head extending away from torso

Neck lengthening

Shoulder blades drawn away from neck

Natural lumbar curve retained

Tailbone extending away from torso

Legs extending away from torso

Ankles, knees, and hips in alignment

Feet hip-distance apart

Forehead resting on back of hands and gaze focused toward floor

Pelvic floor and abdominal muscles engaged to hold lumbar spine in position

Pubic bone imprinting into floor

Make it easier

Put a cushion under your pelvis if your pubic bone or hips are bony and you are uncomfortable when doing the exercise.

LYING ON YOUR SIDE IN NEUTRAL

When you lie on your side in neutral, make sure your ankles, knees, hips, shoulder girdle, and ears are in alignment. Lengthen through the legs. Engage your abdominal muscles to support your spine and contract your pelvic floor muscles to keep your pelvis stable and in alignment.

Extend the arm lying on the floor and rest your head on it. Use your free arm to balance your body by placing the palm of your hand on the floor in front of your chest. Make sure that your top hip is stacked directly over the lower hip and not rotating the pelvis by leaning backward or forward.

Working from this position challenges the core stability muscles of your torso. When breathing in a side-lying position, inhale into the back of the ribcage and as you exhale, pull your navel inward and upward so that your waist appears to lift off the floor. You should be able to see daylight under your waist on the exhale. Focusing on deep breathing in this position will help to improve your balance.

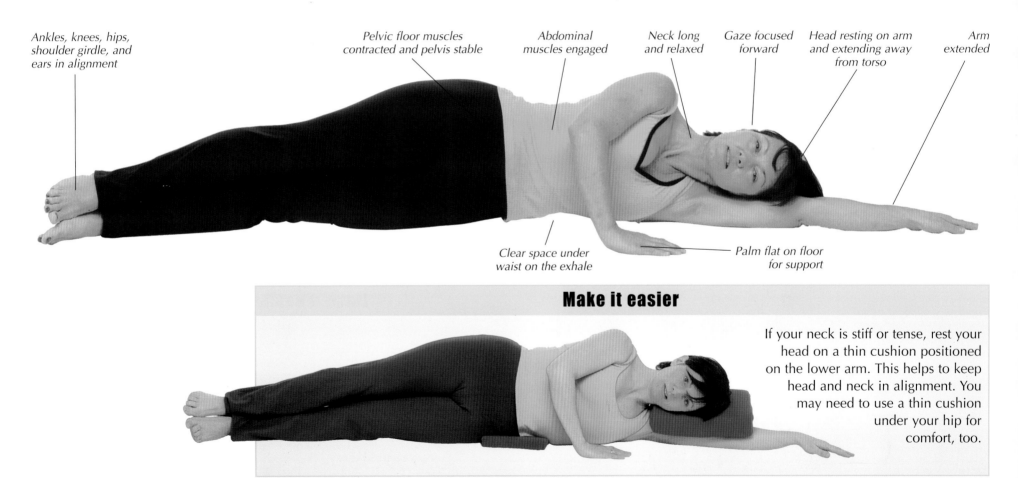

Ankles, knees, hips, shoulder girdle, and ears in alignment

Pelvic floor muscles contracted and pelvis stable

Abdominal muscles engaged

Neck long and relaxed

Gaze focused forward

Head resting on arm and extending away from torso

Arm extended

Clear space under waist on the exhale

Palm flat on floor for support

Make it easier

If your neck is stiff or tense, rest your head on a thin cushion positioned on the lower arm. This helps to keep head and neck in alignment. You may need to use a thin cushion under your hip for comfort, too.

KNEELING ON ALL FOURS IN NEUTRAL

To find neutral spine when kneeling on all fours, first make sure your knees and ankles are hip-distance apart. Your knees should be directly under your hips, creating a line from the knee to the hip joint that is perpendicular to the floor.

Place your palms flat on the floor with fingers pointing forward. Wrists, elbows, and arms should be directly below your shoulders.

Extend your tailbone backward, away from your torso. Make sure your pubic bone and hipbones are in alignment. Engage your pelvic floor and abdominal muscles to maintain your lumbar spine in neutral without over-exaggerating the curve.

Extend your chest forward, drawing the top of your ribcage away from your hips. This will help to prevent exaggerating the thoracic curve. Draw your shoulder blades down the back, away from your neck.

Lengthen your neck muscles by drawing your chin in and extending the top of your head forward. Focus your gaze toward the floor.

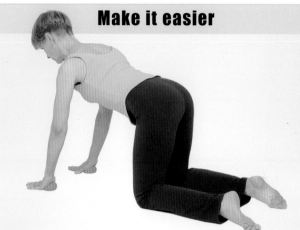

Make it easier

If your wrists feel uncomfortable when the palms are flat on the floor or you have carpel tunnel syndrome, raise your palms by putting a soft, foam, tennis-size ball under each hand.

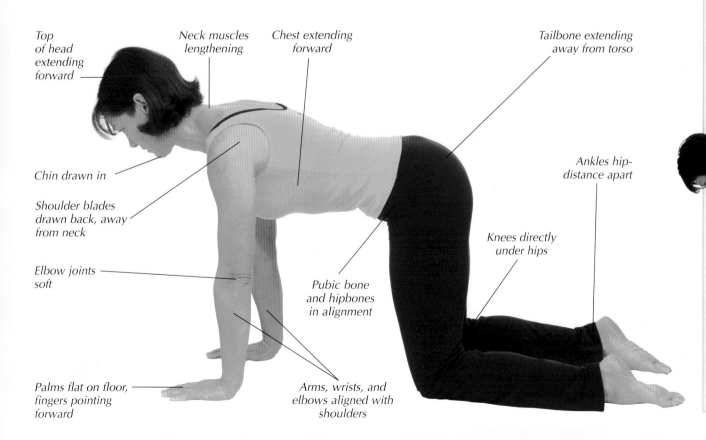

Top of head extending forward

Neck muscles lengthening

Chest extending forward

Tailbone extending away from torso

Chin drawn in

Shoulder blades drawn back, away from neck

Elbow joints soft

Pubic bone and hipbones in alignment

Knees directly under hips

Ankles hip-distance apart

Palms flat on floor, fingers pointing forward

Arms, wrists, and elbows aligned with shoulders

You may find that exercising in an all fours position causes discomfort in the knees. If so, put a thin cushion under them.

SITTING IN NEUTRAL

Sitting in neutral is uncomfortable for many people. Weak back muscles and tight hamstrings that pull the pelvis out of alignment cause this discomfort. Back muscles become weak because we rely on chairs for support; we no longer use our back muscles to keep us upright in a sitting position.

To sit in neutral, first sit on the floor with your legs outstretched. Make sure your hipbones are lined up directly over the sitz bones. Your sitz bones should imprint into the floor.

Lengthen up through your spine, aligning your shoulders directly over your hips. Float your chest upward, without leaning back. Let your shoulders relax backward and down in alignment with your hips.

Align your head over your shoulders and extend your neck. Feel your neck lifting upward from the top of your head.

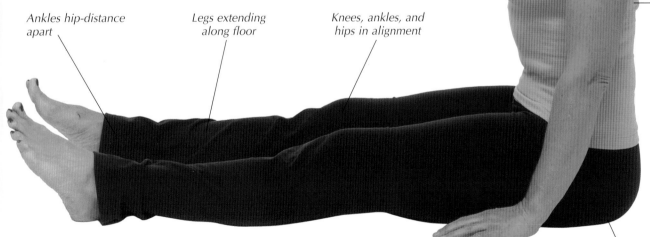

Gaze focused forward

Head lifting from top

Neck extending upward

Shoulders drawn down and aligned with hips

Spine upright and in neutral with natural spinal curves in place

Ankles hip-distance apart

Legs extending along floor

Knees, ankles, and hips in alignment

Sitz bones (the points of the pelvis) imprinting into floor

Sitz bones

If you are not sure where your sitz bones are, pull the cheeks of your buttocks outward so you can feel the two bony points of your pelvis on the floor.

Make it easier

If sitting in neutral with your legs extended feels uncomfortable, place a large, firm cushion under your buttocks to raise you up. You can also bend your knees if necessary to relieve any tightness in the hamstrings.

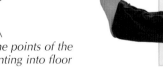

CHAPTER

3

Good
Breathing

About good breathing

In everyday life we take breathing for granted. We all know we need to breathe to stay alive, but most of us are unaware of the importance of breathing correctly.

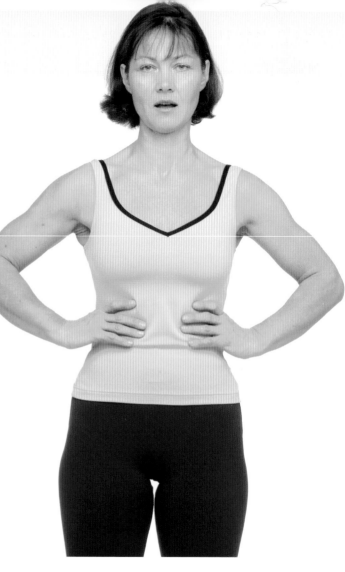

Most people breathe quite shallowly and rarely use the full capacity of their lungs. As a result they have poor cardiovascular fitness. When you breathe, you fill your lungs with air. The oxygen in the air moves from your lungs into your blood stream. The blood then carries the oxygen around the body and to the vital organs, which need plenty of oxygen to function efficiently.

When you breathe more deeply than normal, you draw more oxygen into your lungs. This fires up your metabolism, energizing your muscles and calming your senses. Deep breathing also helps to clear your mind and improve mental focus. That is why people are often advised take a deep breath before attempting an important task.

Breathing and the Pilates method

Good breathing technique plays an integral role in the Pilates method. Deep, slow breathing helps to relax the muscles. When muscles are relaxed, they become more pliable, function more efficiently, and therefore gain a far greater benefit from the exercises. Correct breathing technique is also the key to executing Pilates exercises well. Most exercises are performed in a slow, controlled manner, and breathing governs the speed at which you do the exercise. Slowing down joint movement so that it follows the rhythm of a slow breath gives you time to concentrate on controlling the movement and maximizes the effort your muscles make. This gives you the maximum benefit from a simple stretch or extension.

Before practicing Pilates exercises, you must first learn how to breathe correctly. In Pilates you breathe by slowly expanding and contracting your lungs—moving only your ribcage and keeping the rest of your body still. To do this, you need to expand your ribcage sideways and backward on the inhale and close the ribcage, engage the pelvic floor muscles, and pull the navel in and up as you exhale. This movement of the ribcage activates the muscles between your ribs, called the intercostals, and those around your thoracic spine at the back of your ribcage. Mobilizing the muscles in this way helps to make you aware of the deeper muscles of the torso that are connected to the spine. It also stretches and strengthens the muscles, easing away stiffness and tension in the back and neck.

Choose a peaceful and warm place in which to practice so you can focus on your breathing in comfort. To check that your ribcage is moving in the correct way, place your fingertips on the apex of the ribcage (where it divides at the bottom of the ribs) and feel the apex close on the exhale and open on the inhale. It will take practice and a little patience, but gradually breathing correctly will feel natural and you will become aware of its importance when exercising.

Timing the breath

As you practice your breathing, count slowly and steadily as you breathe in and out to see how long you take for each. Try to build up to a count of five for the inhale and five for the exhale. Most movements in Pilates are done at a slow speed and are linked to the speed of the breath.

Correct ribcage breathing

1 Stand in the neutral spine position with your shoulders relaxed. Place your hands around the base of your ribcage, thumbs to the back and fingers spread around the front. Start breathing normally and focus your mind on how you breathe. Then relax your jawline so that your mouth is slightly open and your face is relaxed. **Inhale slowly and deeply through your nose,** expanding your ribcage sideways and backward. You should feel your ribcage expand into your hands. When breathing in, try not to lift your shoulders—isolate the movement to the ribcage area only.

2 Exhale slowly and deeply through your mouth, closing your ribcage by drawing the front of the ribcage in and down and letting your chest relax (or "soften"). You should feel your ribs shrink away from your hands. When you can feel this movement, no matter how subtle, it means that the intercostal muscles between your ribs are being activated. Isolate the movement to the ribcage area only. Engage your pelvic floor muscles and activate your transversus muscle (the deep core stabilizing muscle) by pulling your navel in and up as you exhale.

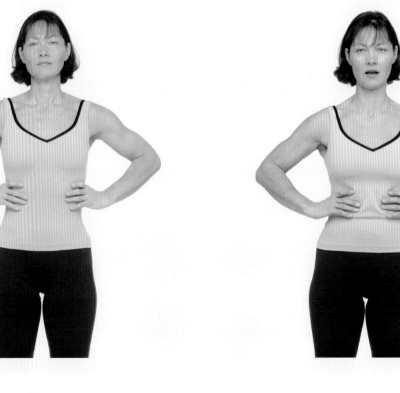

PILATES BREATHING EXERCISE

If you are new to Pilates, think of this as your very first exercise using Pilates techniques. It links deep breathing with standing in neutral spine. Although no joints are moved, your core stability muscles will be activated as you learn to control deep breathing while at the same time maintaining a good posture. This breathing technique is called ribcage breathing.

Practice this exercise as often as you can throughout the day. Even if you concentrate on just this one exercise for several weeks, you will not be wasting your time. Practicing it will strengthen your intercostal and abdominal muscles. Collectively these muscles create your core stability. Repetition of deep breathing will also flatten your stomach, greatly improve your lung capacity, benefit cardiovascular fitness, and help you to relax.

The beauty of the exercise, aside from the physical benefits, is the fact that you can do it any time, anywhere. It can also be practiced in the other neutral spine positions (see page 29).

On the exhale...

- Close the ribcage, softening down through the breastbone and closing the apex of the ribcage.

- Draw your navel inward and upward as your breastbone softens so that you can connect to your center where your transversus muscle (or powerhouse!) is located. Do not push your belly out.

- Engage your pelvic floor muscles by contracting up through the vagina and/or anus without squeezing the buttocks or moving the pelvis.

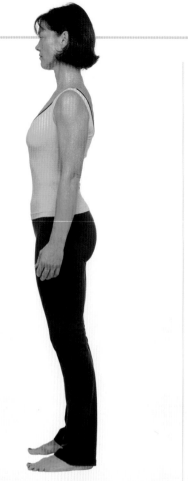

1 Stand in neutral spine with your arms relaxed at your sides; your ankles, hips, and shoulders aligned; your shoulders relaxed; and your neck extended (see page 19 for more about standing in neutral). A bad posture will prevent you from fully opening your ribcage. Relax in this position before you start to concentrate on deep breathing.

2 Inhale slowly and deeply through your nose, expanding your ribcage sideways and backward. As you take this slow, deep breath, maintain your neutral spine position with its natural curves. Keeping your shoulders still, move only your ribcage. You should be feeling very stable and grounded.

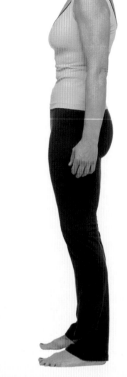

3 Exhale slowly and deeply through the mouth, drawing the front of your ribcage in and down. Mobilize your abdominal muscles by pulling the navel in, drawing it up toward the ribcage, and engaging your pelvic floor muscles. Think of flattening and lengthening the abdominal wall. Keep your shoulders still and relaxed.

Repeat steps 2 and 3 five times in a slow, rhythmic manner.

Ribcage breathing is the same whether you are doing Pilates exercises lying on your back, lying on your front, on all fours, or seated. However, you will feel the slow expansion and slow closing of the ribcage slightly differently in each position.

Remember, you must be in the neutral spine position in order to breathe properly. If you are not, you will not be able to open your ribcage fully. To review the correct neutral spine positions, refer back to Chapter 2.

Everyday breathing

Practice ribcage breathing every day, wherever and whenever you can—driving your car, standing at the checkout, peeling potatoes. Mental focus and repetition will help your breathing technique become natural. Try to slow down your breathing and deepen it. Feel your ribcage expand and close. On the exhale, feel the abdominal muscles drawing inward and upward, flattening and lengthening the abdominal wall. Engage your pelvic floor muscles.

In all neutral positions

- Breathe in through your nose and out through your mouth—slowly, deeply, and in a controlled rhythm.
- Keep your pelvis and spine in their neutral positions.
- Keep your shoulders relaxed.
- **On the inhale,** expand the ribcage sideways and backward.
- **On the exhale,** close the ribcage, engage pelvic floor and abdominal muscles, and draw the navel in and up.

On your back

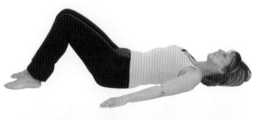

Lying on your back in neutral (see page 20) is the best way to feel the correct Pilates breathing technique. On the inhale, as your ribcage expands sideways and backward, you should feel the back of the ribs imprinting deeper into the floor. Do not move your shoulders when breathing; keep them stable and relaxed on the floor. (This is a good exercise for women after giving birth.)

On your front

Lie on your front in neutral (see page 21). Keep your shoulders, head, and neck completely relaxed when breathing in this position. As you exhale, pull your navel off the floor and toward your spine. The triangle of your pubic bone and hipbones should be imprinting into the floor, creating a small cavity under your belly. When you inhale, keep the abdominal muscles engaged so that your belly does not collapse onto the floor, pulling your pelvis out of alignment.

On all fours

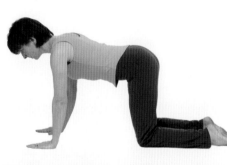

Kneel on all fours in neutral (see page 23), and make sure that your knees are directly under your hips. When inhaling, use the intercostal muscles between your ribs to expand your ribcage sideways and backward. When you close the front of the ribcage on the exhale, use your abdominal muscles to draw the navel in toward the spine and up toward the neck.

Seated

Sit in neutral (see page 24). As this is a more difficult position to maintain, you may prefer to sit on a firm cushion, bend your knees, or sit with your back against the wall when practicing deep breathing. Breathing when seated in neutral should feel similar to breathing in the standing position, but it will require more effort to keep your spine and pelvis in neutral at the same time.

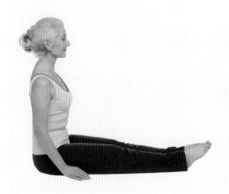

Once you have mastered the various neutral spine positions and practiced ribcage breathing, you are ready to move and breathe at the same time!

The Pelvic Rock is an ideal exercise for experimenting. It is a fairly easy movement that most people can manage, even those with restricted mobility. Designed to mobilize the lumbar and pelvic area of the spine, it is often practiced to relieve discomfort in the lower back. The slow, continuous motion of the exercise should be like a rocking chair that is rocking smoothly and evenly, back and forth with the breath.

The more you have practiced deep ribcage breathing in neutral spine, the easier it will be to add movement. The principle of linking movement and breath is the same for all Pilates exercises, so by practicing with this simple movement, you will begin to understand the principles of all Pilates movements.

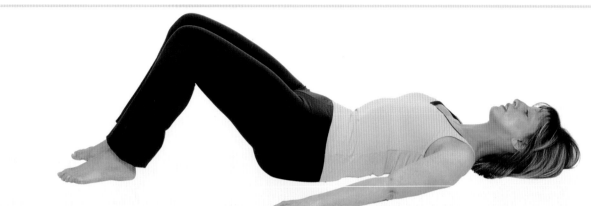

1 Lie in neutral spine position, with your knees bent and hip-distance apart, and relax. Start your deep breathing as explained on page 29. **Inhale** and **exhale** a few times until you feel you are breathing in a slow, controlled way, ending with an exhalation. **Inhale to prepare for your first movement**.

Exhale through your mouth in the slow, controlled rhythm that you have established.
In time with your exhalation, slowly tilt your pubic bone toward your ribs so that the lumbar spine (the lower back) sinks gently into the floor. Let the breathing control the speed of the movement.

Ribcage breathing

- Ribcage breathing activates the intercostal muscles, the deep muscles of the torso, and the pelvic floor muscles—muscles that create your core stability.

- In Pilates you usually exhale on the extension or effort of a movement.

- The inhale is often the preparation for a movement or occurs on the release back to the starting position.

2 Inhale through your nose in the slow, controlled breathing rhythm that you have established.
In time with your slow inhalation, slowly extend your pubic bone away from your ribs, arching your lower back away from the floor, back into neutral spine.

Repeat 4–6 times, concentrating on linking each upward tilt of the pelvis with an exhalation and each return to neutral with an inhalation.

Getting Started

CHAPTER 4

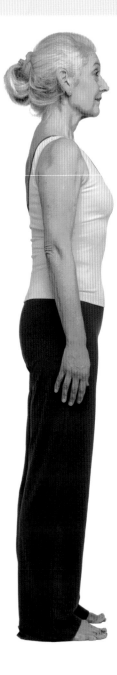

This chapter introduces you to a series of standing exercises that will mobilize and warm up your joints and muscles. It is important to warm up your body before you move on to the mat work. These exercises also help to prepare you mentally and physically for some of the more strenuous exercises in later chapters.

Whether you have just woken up in the morning or have spent a long day standing, sitting, carrying, or lifting, always take a few minutes to prepare for your Pilates exercises. Time spent correcting your posture and focusing on your breathing improves your technique and mental focus.

First, check your postural alignment by going through the checklist for standing in neutral (see right). Then follow the exercises on the next page to make sure your pelvis and head are correctly aligned.

Finally, practice ribcage breathing, as explained on page 33, before moving into the warm-up exercises in this chapter.

Standing in neutral

- Stand with your feet together, then turn your toes outward, leaving your heels and legs together.

- Line up your heels with your toes so that your ankles, knees, and hips are in alignment.

- Make sure that your feet do not roll outward or inward and that your body weight is evenly distributed between the ball and the heel of each foot.

- Check that your knees are slightly bent (soft), facing front, and not rolling inward.

- Line up your pelvis (see page 33).

- Extend your tailbone toward the floor, keeping your buttocks relaxed.

- Make sure that your lumbar spine above your pelvis retains its natural concave curve. Lift your breastbone toward the ceiling and let your shoulders relax downward. To help lengthen your torso, imagine that a piece of string is attached to your breastbone and is being gently pulled upward.

- Keep your shoulder girdle, which sits on top of the ribcage, relaxed back and down so that your shoulder joints are in alignment with your hips, knees, and ankles.

- Keep your ribcage area—the cylinder containing the vital organs—in an open and lengthened position so the organs are not compressed.

- Align your head over your shoulders and feel that you are lifting from the top of your head.

Moving your pelvis into neutral

Remember how to move your pelvis and head into alignment. This is also covered on page 18 in Chapter 2, but as you learn Pilates, you must go over and over this until it becomes an automatic part of your routine—and of your daily life.

To check that your pelvis is in alignment, place your fingertips over your pubic bone and the heels of your hands over your hipbones, making a V-shape.

Your hands should form a level triangle perpendicular to the floor. If they aren't, use the simple exercise at the right to position your pelvis correctly. Stand in the neutral spine position with your fingertips in place. Tilt your pelvis as far forward as you can, then as far back. Next, move into a position midway between these two extremes. Your pelvis should now be in neutral with your hands creating a level triangle.

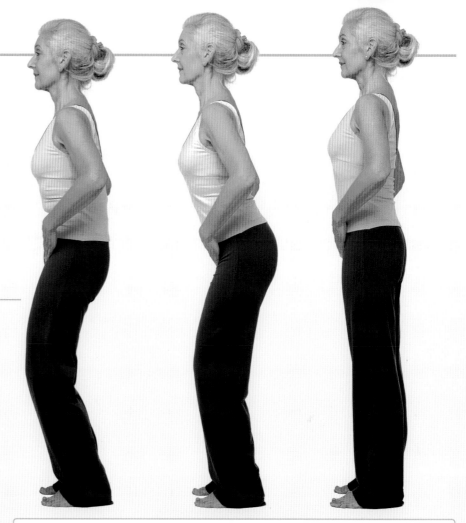

Aligning your head

Your head should be aligned over your shoulders, with your chin pulled back and tucked in toward your neck and your gaze focusing forward. To achieve the correct alignment, first stand in position and jut your chin forward. Then draw your chin in and back so that your neck is lengthening and you feel that you are lifting from the top of your head, which is directly above your shoulders.

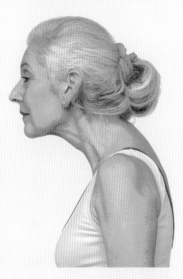
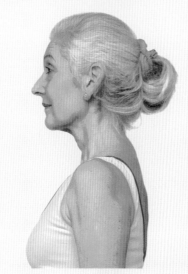

Breathing practice

Once you have positioned yourself correctly in a well-aligned standing posture, practice the deep, slow, ribcage breathing explained here. This practice will help you become more aware of how to expand the back of your ribcage on the inhalation during your exercises. It will also establish the slow, rhythmic pace of your movements.

- **As you inhale,** expand your ribcage sideways and backward.

- **As you exhale,** engage your pelvic floor muscles, draw your navel inward toward your spine and upward, and close the front of your ribcage without moving your spine or pelvis.

Many people hold tension in the neck. This can result in tight, weak muscles in this area that often lead to headaches. The Cervical Nod is a subtle but effective exercise. It will make you more aware of your neck muscles and the movement that takes place between the atlas—the first cervical vertebra at the very top of your spine—and the base of your head.

Gentle movement in this area will release tension and help to lengthen and strengthen your neck muscles. It is a good warm-up exercise before you move into exercises on the mat.

Correct practice

- Keep your shoulders still as your head rolls down.

- Do not force your head down.

- Visualize the vertebra moving as you lower your head and roll it back up.

- Roll your head up and down in time with your deep ribcage breathing.

1 Stand in neutral.
As you inhale, slowly draw your chin inward and down toward the chest, only moving the first cervical vertebra.

2 **As you exhale,** slowly roll your head back up into alignment with your shoulders, feeling your neck muscles lengthen.

Repeat 4 times in a smooth, rolling movement.

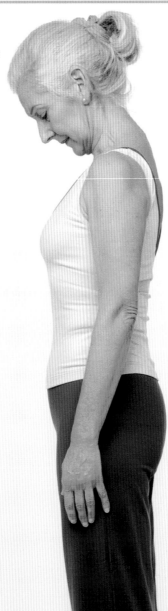

This simple standing exercise releases tension from the neck and shoulders. Use it as part of your warm-up to gently mobilize your shoulders and upper spine. You can practice the exercise at any time, sitting or standing, when you are tense or feel a headache coming on.

As with all Pilates exercises, keep the movement flowing in time with your slow, deep breathing.

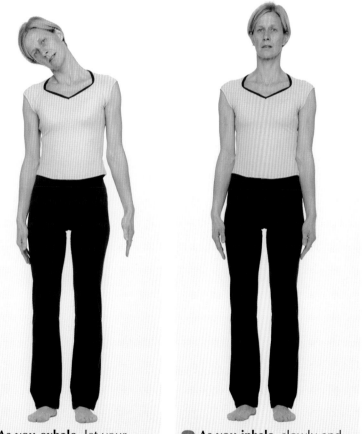

1 Standing or sitting in a good posture, **inhale**.

2 **As you exhale,** let your head tilt to the right side, with your ear slowly lowering to your shoulder. Keep both shoulders stable and do not allow the opposite shoulder to lift.

3 **As you inhale,** slowly and gently lift your head back into alignment.

4 **As you exhale,** let your head gently tilt to the left side. **As you inhale,** slowly return your head to the center.

Repeat twice on each side alternately.

To relieve neck pain

This gentle neck stretch can be done at any time to help relieve headaches or neck tension.

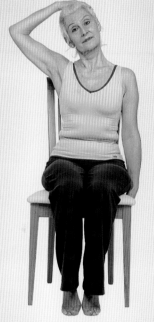

Sitting upright, hold the edge of the chair with your left hand. Place the right hand over your head. **Inhale.**
As you exhale, tilt the head to the right, lengthening the neck muscles. Applying minimal pressure with your hand, breathe slowly in this position for 15 seconds. Repeat on the other side.

The Knee Bends exercise can easily be seen as purely a bend and stretch of your knees. But, in fact, it has many more benefits. First, it helps you develop correct foot placement and correct alignment of the ankle, knee, and hip joints when bending and stretching. It also engages the pelvic floor muscles, increasing your awareness of the importance of the core stability muscles. These muscles hold your torso in a good posture while your legs are moving.

Correct practice

- Check your correct foot placement and do not let your feet roll in or out.

- Keep your shoulders over your hips as your knees bend and as you straighten them.

- Do not lock your knee joints as you straighten your legs.

- Do not clench your buttocks.

- Keep your shoulders and neck relaxed and in the correct alignment.

- Focus on your slow, deep, ribcage breathing and move in time with it.

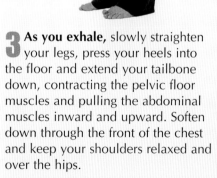

1 Stand in neutral and relax.

2 As you inhale, slowly bend your knees, keeping your kneecaps facing forward. Go as low as you can without lifting your heels off the floor. Allow your hip flexors to relax as you bend your knees so that your pelvis stays in neutral and your shoulders remain over your hips. Do not allow your pelvis to tilt.

3 As you exhale, slowly straighten your legs, press your heels into the floor and extend your tailbone down, contracting the pelvic floor muscles and pulling the abdominal muscles inward and upward. Soften down through the front of the chest and keep your shoulders relaxed and over the hips.

Repeat 6 times.

Rocking your pelvis helps you find the correct—neutral—position for your pelvis and mobilizes the lumbar spine.

Correct pelvic alignment is fundamental to maintaining a neutral spine and misalignment can cause lower-back pain and hip-joint problems.

To line up the pelvis, find your tailbone, technically known as the coccyx—the last vertebrae at the bottom of the spine. Concentrate on extending your tailbone toward the floor, keeping your buttocks relaxed. The pubic bone and the hipbones should be in alignment with each other, creating a flat triangle perpendicular to the floor.

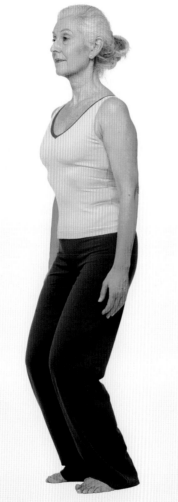

1 Stand in neutral with your pubic bone and hipbones in alignment, then bend your knees slightly to prepare to move into the exercise.

2 **As you inhale,** slowly tilt your pelvis as far forward as you can. (When performing this exercise, you may find it easier if you can feel your pelvis move, so position your hands as explained on page 33.)

3 **As you exhale,** slowly tilt your pelvis as far back as you can. Keep the movement smoothly flowing in a rocking motion as you tilt forward and back.

Repeat 6–8 times.

This standing Half Roll-Down exercise focuses on mobilizing and flexing the upper part of the spine, called the thoracic spine. To help you move correctly and with your breathing, imagine your spine is like a string of pearls and each vertebra or pearl is moving individually as you roll down and up.

Use the Half Roll-Down to warm up the upper part of your spine before attempting the Full Roll-Down.

1 Stand in neutral, with your body relaxed and in correct alignment. **As you inhale,** slowly curl your head forward, following with your neck and shoulders.

2 **As you exhale,** gently and smoothly roll down through each vertebra in the upper back and then through the vertebrae in the back of the ribcage until your shoulders are level with your waist. Make sure your head, neck, and shoulders are completely relaxed. Keep your knees, hips, and ankles in alignment so that you are not sitting back into your hips.

3 **As you inhale,** start uncurling through each vertebra in the back of the ribcage and continue to uncurl smoothly up through the vertebrae of the upper back.

4 **Start exhaling** as your shoulders come into place followed by the neck. **Still on the exhale,** bring your head up into alignment so you are once again in the neutral spine position.

Repeat 3 times in a flowing movement.

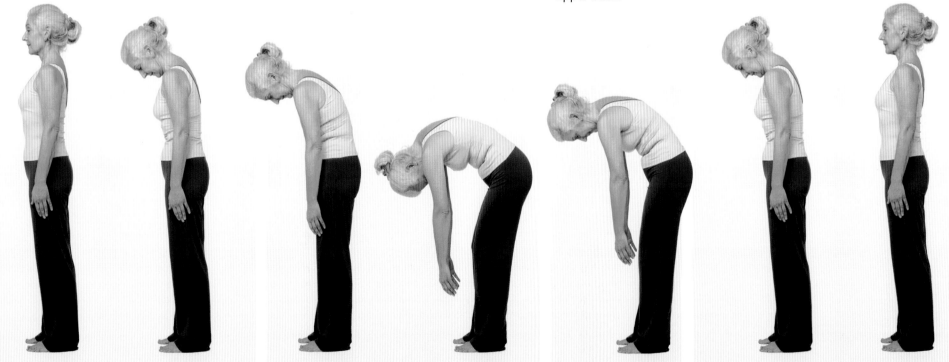

FULL ROLL-DOWN—SPINE MOBILITY

Now you are ready to mobilize and flex the whole spine. As with the Half Roll-Down, visualizing the movement of each vertebra, one at a time, will help you move correctly with your breathing. Again, imagine that your spine is like a string of pearls and each vertebra or pearl is moving individually as you roll down and up.

Make sure you bend your knees as your shoulders pass the waist and as you are coming up from the lowest position.

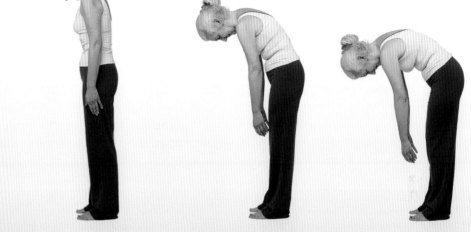

1 Stand in neutral. **As you inhale,** curl your head forward, followed by your neck and shoulders, and slowly roll down through the vertebrae of the upper back. **Still on the inhale,** keep on gently rolling down to waist level.

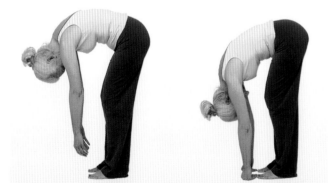

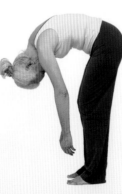

2 Continue rolling down, **exhaling as you pass waist level** and bending your knees slightly to take you as far down as you can go without forcing your body. Make sure your head, neck, shoulders, and arms are completely relaxed. Keep your knees, hips, and ankles in alignment so you are not sitting back into your hips.

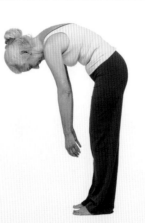

3 Keep the movement flowing. **As you inhale,** start smoothly uncurling, dropping your tailbone toward the floor and uncurling upward through the lower back.

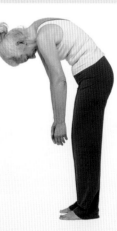

4 As your shoulders come up past the waist, **exhale** to uncurl through the upper back and neck. Then bring your head up into alignment.

Repeat 4–6 times in a smooth, flowing movement.

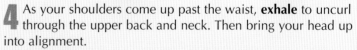

FULL ROLL-DOWN IN FOCUS

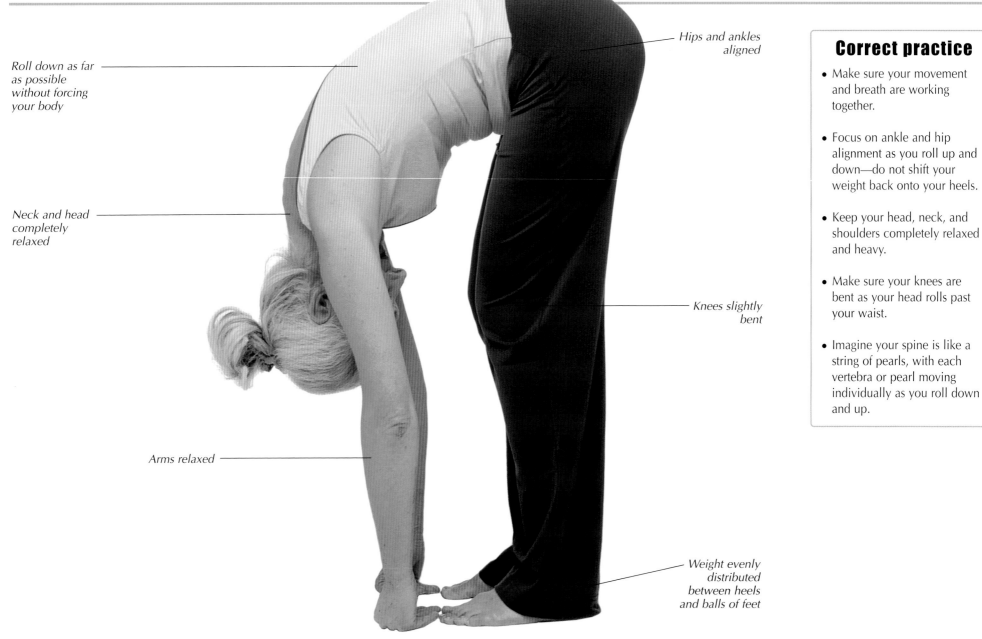

Roll down as far as possible without forcing your body

Neck and head completely relaxed

Arms relaxed

Hips and ankles aligned

Knees slightly bent

Weight evenly distributed between heels and balls of feet

Correct practice

- Make sure your movement and breath are working together.

- Focus on ankle and hip alignment as you roll up and down—do not shift your weight back onto your heels.

- Keep your head, neck, and shoulders completely relaxed and heavy.

- Make sure your knees are bent as your head rolls past your waist.

- Imagine your spine is like a string of pearls, with each vertebra or pearl moving individually as you roll down and up.

The Lateral Stretch will increase the range of movement through your back muscles, improving your back's flexibility. This exercise not only feels great to do, but it also releases tight muscles in the lower back.

While holding the stretch in this exercise, rotate your neck to make yourself aware of the correct head placement and to release tension in your neck and shoulders.

CAUTION: If you have a severe back problem, avoid this exercise.

1 Stand in neutral.

2 As you inhale, slowly float your right arm up toward the ceiling until it is above your head, making sure your pelvis remains in neutral. Keep your right shoulder in place and turn your palm toward you as your hand passes your shoulder.

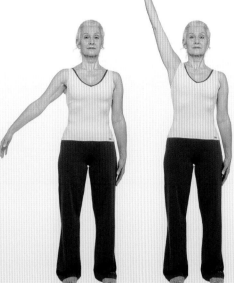

3 As you exhale, gently slide your left hand down the side of your body as your ribcage lifts and lengthens from the waist over to the left. Let your head, neck, and shoulders relax completely and keep your weight centered so that your feet are taking your body weight evenly.

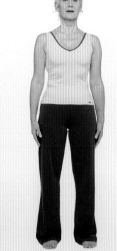

4 As you inhale, gently rotate your head and look up to your palm. Keep your arm lengthening, fingers relaxed, and wrist aligned with the forearm.

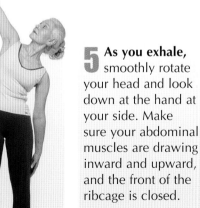

5 As you exhale, smoothly rotate your head and look down at the hand at your side. Make sure your abdominal muscles are drawing inward and upward, and the front of the ribcage is closed.

6 As you inhale, look back up into your palm. Keep your right shoulder down and relaxed.

7 As you exhale, lift your torso back up to an upright position and allow your arm to float back down to your side.

Repeat on the other side.

Arm lengthening upward and fingers relaxed

Arm lifted only as far up as flexibility allows

Right shoulder kept down as arm lifts

Ribcage lifting and lengthening laterally from waist

Head rotating up on inhale and down on exhale

Shoulder stable and shoulder blades drawing down

Abdominal muscles pulling inward and upward

Pelvis in neutral and weight evenly distributed over both hips

Feet taking weight evenly

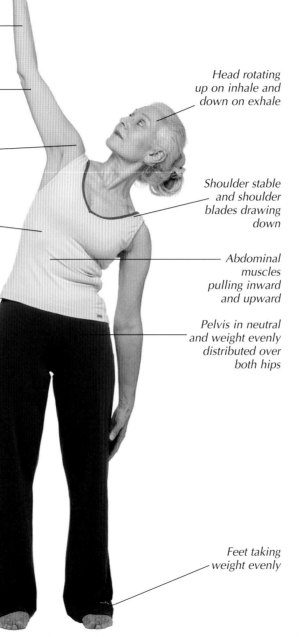

Correct practice

- Check neutral alignment before you begin.

- Keep your shoulders stable and your shoulder blades drawing down as your arm lifts.

- Lengthen up from the waist into the lateral stretch.

- Rotate your neck to look at the palm of your raised hand.

- Retain pelvic alignment.

- Keep the big toe and little toe of each foot on the floor.

Good alignment

As you lengthen and stretch to the side, make sure that your body stays in alignment. Do not roll forward from the hip.

Common mistake

As you stretch over to one side, try not to shift your weight onto the opposite leg. And when your arm is lifting, try not to let your shoulder rise toward your ear.

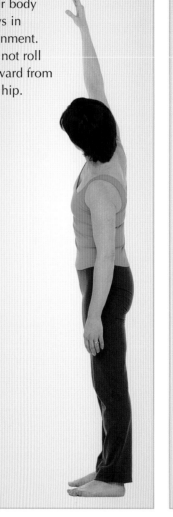

Once you are confident that you can do the Pilates exercises in this chapter, you can use them together as a gentle 5–10-minute exercise routine or as a warm-up for other, more strenuous, routines in the book.

Follow the sequence of the exercises as they are shown here and remember to move slowly, following the even rhythm of your deep breathing. Do not stop between exercises, but keep the movements flowing from one exercise to the next, as if you are performing a gentle, choreographed dance.

Cervical Nod—Standing (page 34)

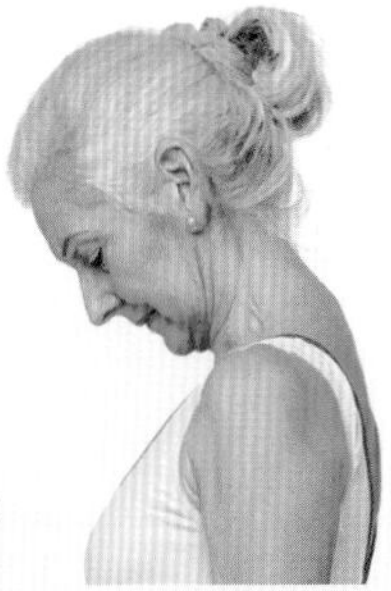

1 **Inhale**—draw chin inward and down.

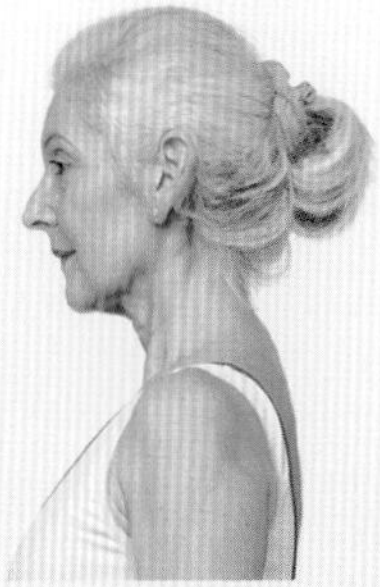

2 **Exhale**—release back to neutral.

Repeat 4 times.

Knee Bends (page 36)

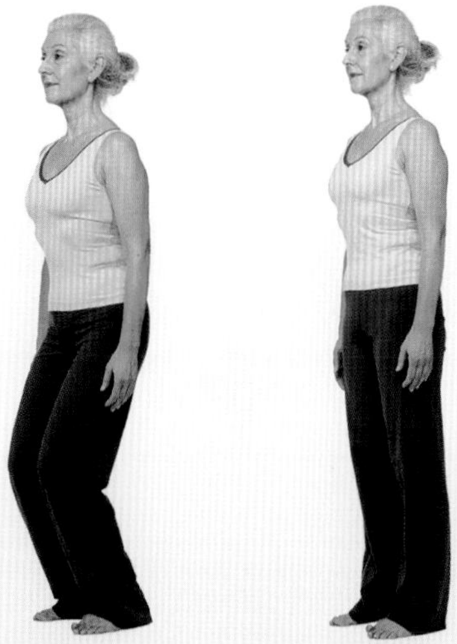

1 **Inhale**—bend knees.

2 **Exhale**—straighten legs.

Repeat 4 times.

Pelvic Rock (page 37)

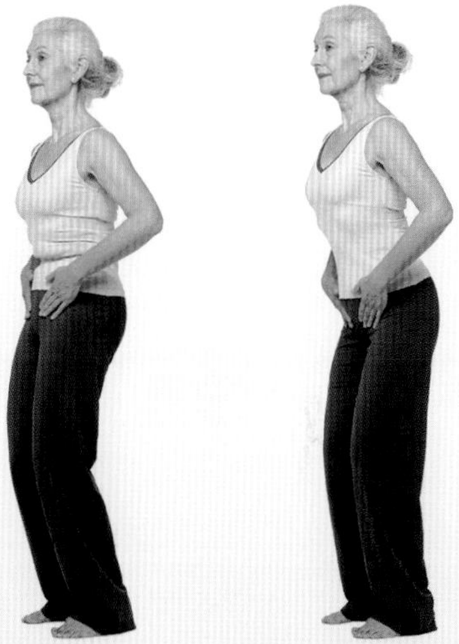

1 **Inhale**—tilt pelvis forward.

2 **Exhale**—tilt pelvis backward.

Repeat 4 times.

Half Roll-Down (page 38)

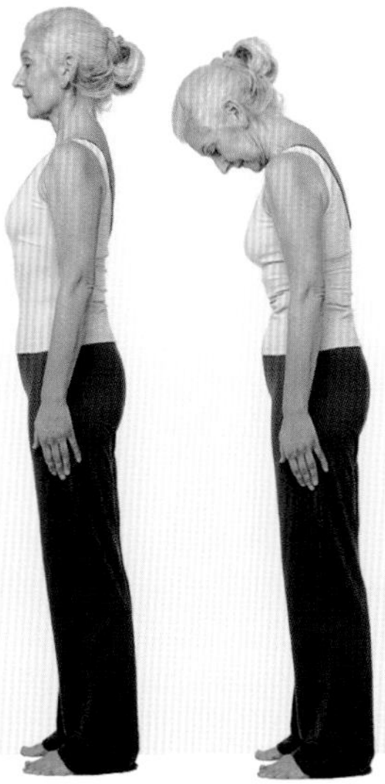

1 **Inhale**—start curling head, neck, and shoulders.

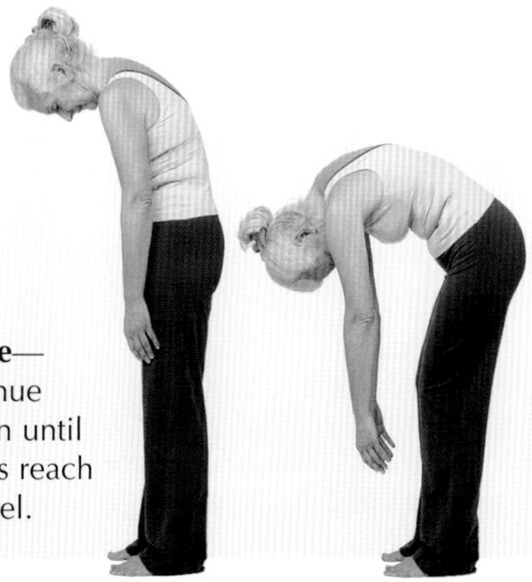

2 **Exhale**—continue roll-down until shoulders reach waist level.

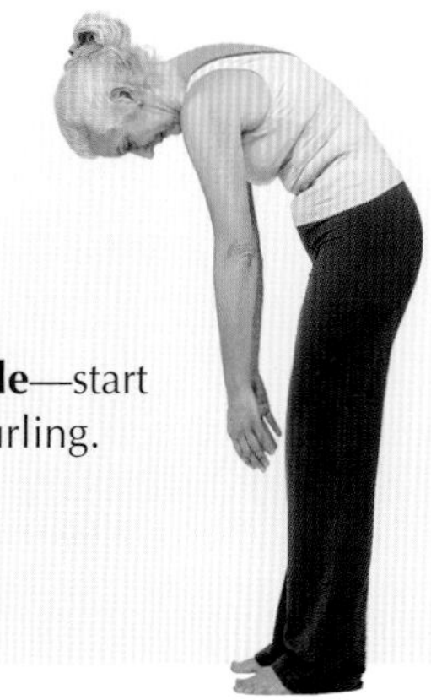

3 **Inhale**—start uncurling.

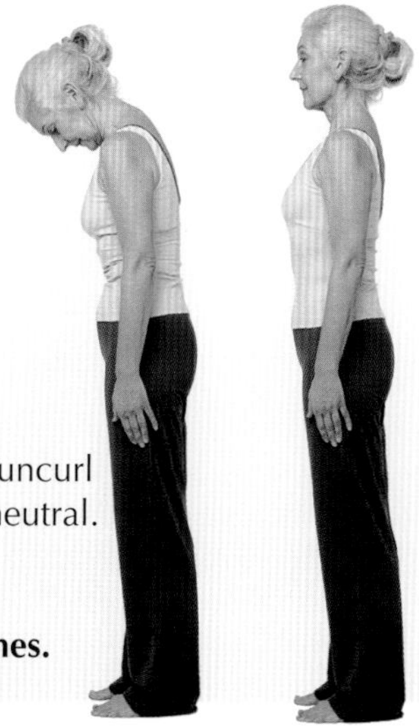

4 **Exhale**—uncurl back to neutral.

Repeat 3 times.

continued on next page

Full Roll-Down (page 39)

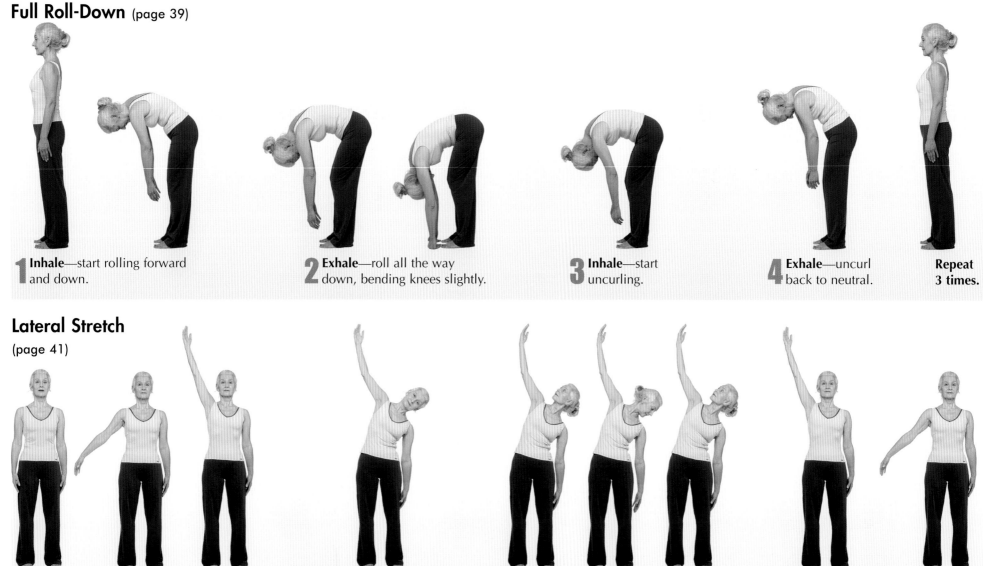

1 Inhale—start rolling forward and down.

2 Exhale—roll all the way down, bending knees slightly.

3 Inhale—start uncurling.

4 Exhale—uncurl back to neutral.

Repeat 3 times.

Lateral Stretch

(page 41)

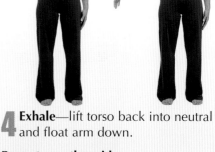

1 Inhale—float right arm up.

2 Exhale—slide left arm down side of body.

3 Inhale—rotate head up.
Exhale—rotate head down.
Inhale—rotate head up.

4 Exhale—lift torso back into neutral and float arm down.

Repeat on other side.

5

Working Your Core Muscles

About your core muscles

The core muscles of your torso are responsible for keeping your spine in neutral alignment. The exercises in this chapter concentrate on mobilizing and maintaining these core muscles.

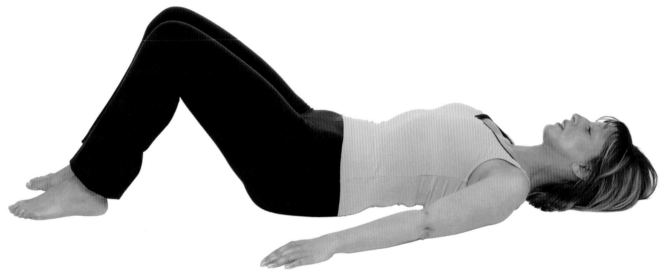

Good spinal alignment helps keep the heaviest parts of your body—the pelvis, ribcage, and head—in balance. Good balance minimizes stress on the joints. If there is any imbalance it will affect your posture, which can lead to pain or injury. For example, if you jut your head forward, your neck muscles will be shortened. This creates tightness in your shoulders and can cause headaches. Or, if you round your shoulders, the front of the ribcage sinks and the chest muscles tighten. This reduces mobility of the intercostal muscles and restricts space for the vital organs.

These exercises work your core muscles. Before you start exercising, review the checklist (see top right) to make sure you are in neutral, and practice your deep breathing.

Lying on your back in neutral

- Lie on your back. Bend your knees and position your legs hip-distance apart so your ankles, knees, and hips are in alignment. Place your feet flat on the floor facing forward in a parallel position, with your toes spread apart.

- Position your pelvis in neutral so that your lower back retains its natural curvature. Make sure your pubic bone and hipbones are level and your tailbone is extending toward your heels. Your sacrum should be imprinting into the floor.

- Imprint your upper spine and shoulder blades into the floor and relax your arms.

- Keep your shoulders relaxed and drawing away from your neck.

- Lengthen through the muscles of the neck and extend the top of your head along the floor.

Breathing practice

- **As you inhale,** feel your shoulders relax and the back of your ribcage imprint deeper into the floor as your ribcage expands sideways and backward.

- **As you exhale,** feel the front of your ribcage drawing in and down. The apex of the ribs should be closing together. At the same time, draw your abdominal muscles inward and upward toward the ribs.

PELVIC ROCK

The Pelvic Rock exercise and Pelvic Clock exercise (page 48) help to gently mobilize the lumbar and pelvic areas of the spine where stiffness, aches, and pains occur, especially after long periods of sitting or standing.

These subtle but effective exercises will improve your pelvic alignment and can be performed at any time throughout your day to relieve discomfort in the lower back.

Remember to breathe deeply and slowly and complete each action in time with either your exhalation or inhalation.

Pelvic alignment

Correct pelvic alignment is vital for a good posture. If the pelvis is tipping forward or backward, it exaggerates the lumbar curve or overflattens it, which restricts movement and can cause lower-back pain. It can also affect the rest of the spine, which will try to compensate for the misalignment.

1 Lie on your back in neutral with your knees bent and hip-distance apart. When you are ready, **inhale** slowly to prepare.

2 **As you exhale,** slowly bring your pelvis up so that your pubic bone tilts toward your navel and the lumbar spine area of the lower back sinks gently into the floor.

3 **As you inhale,** slowly reverse the tilt, extending your pubic bone away from your navel and arching your lower back away from the floor. Keep the movement continuous and flowing— don't stop at either end of either rock.

Repeat 4–6 times.

1 Lie on your back in neutral with knees bent and hip-distance apart.
Inhale slowly to prepare.
As you exhale, slowly bring your pelvis up so that your pubic bone tilts toward your navel.
As you inhale, slowly rock your pelvis to the left side.

2 **As you exhale,** smoothly tilt your pelvis to the right side.
As you inhale, return to neutral.

Repeat 4–6 times.

Correct practice

- Use visualization to help you do this exercise correctly. As you rock your pelvis, imagine that your belly is filled with water (like a goldfish bowl) and that the water is sloshing from one hip to the other.

- Keep the movements continuous and flowing, without stopping at the extreme points of the tilts—like smoothly rocking in a rocking chair. This rocking will mobilize the lower back and help relieve lower-back pain.

Improve your practice

To help focus your mind on the tilting movement in your pelvis and improve your practice, place your fingertips on your hipbones so that you can feel your pelvis tilting.

Keep your shoulders and upper back imprinting into the floor. Make sure your shoulders remain relaxed throughout.

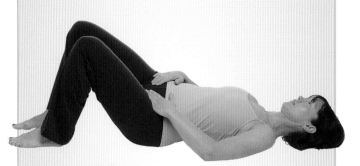

Inhale to prepare. **As you exhale,** slowly lift one hipbone.

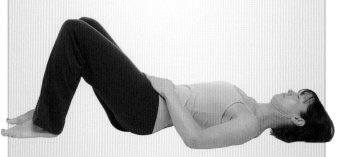

Inhale and **exhale** as you slowly rock from side to side.

THE BRIDGE

The Bridge is an excellent exercise for mobilizing the spine. It also gently lengthens the muscles of the back, which relieves pressure on vertebrae that may have become compressed from long periods of sitting and standing.

By working the deep muscles connected to the vertebrae, this exercise helps you gain control over the movement of each section of your spine.

Your breathing and the contraction of the abdominal muscles control the movement. Do the exercise smoothly, working up and down the spine. One at at time, peel the vertebrae off the floor as you lift your back. As you roll down, press each vertebra down in sequence.

Performing the Bridge feels especially good if your back is aching after an active day.

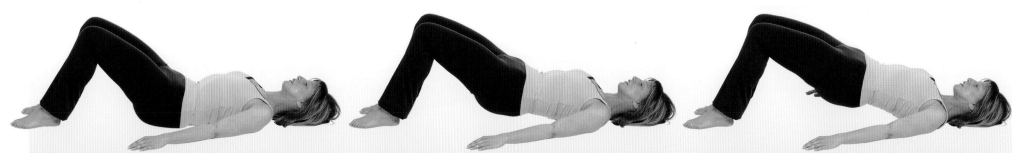

1 Lie on your back in neutral with your knees bent. **Inhale** slowly to prepare.

2 **As you exhale,** bring your pelvis up so that your pubic bone tilts toward your navel. **While still exhaling,** continue smoothly peeling the vertebrae off

the floor one at a time until your body is resting on your shoulder blades. As you curl up, stop your knees from rolling out by engaging the inner thighs and pressing

down through your feet. In the lifted position, the chest, hips, and the tips of your knees should be aligned and the abdominal muscles should be flat or concave.

3 **Inhale** slowly while resting on your shoulder blades, expanding the back of your ribcage.

4 **As you exhale,** work back down through the spine, imprinting one vertebra at a time into the floor until the tailbone touches down.

Repeat 4–6 times slowly in a continuous movement.

Correct practice

- Keep your arms lengthening along the floor and your shoulders relaxed.

- Make sure that your hips lift only to the point where the knees, hips, and shoulders are in alignment and the abdominal muscles are concave. If you raise your hips too high, your head will slide backward.

THE BRIDGE IN FOCUS

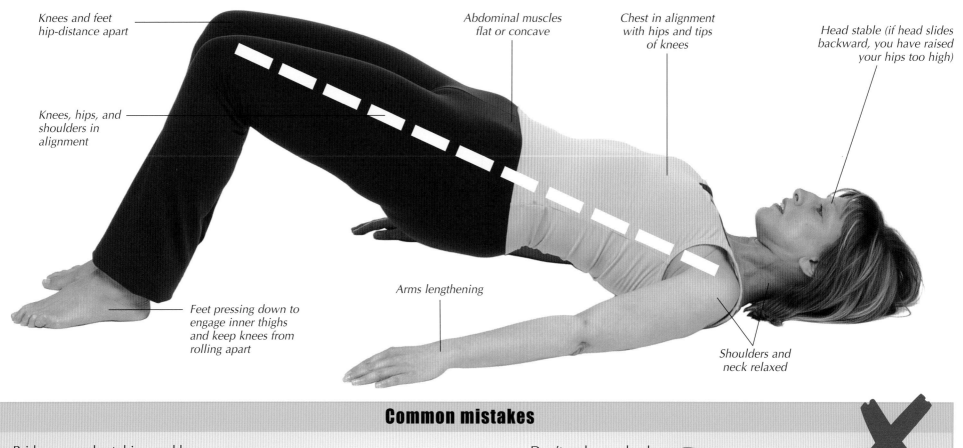

Knees and feet hip-distance apart

Knees, hips, and shoulders in alignment

Feet pressing down to engage inner thighs and keep knees from rolling apart

Abdominal muscles flat or concave

Chest in alignment with hips and tips of knees

Head stable (if head slides backward, you have raised your hips too high)

Arms lengthening

Shoulders and neck relaxed

Common mistakes

In the Bridge, your chest, hips, and knee tips should be aligned, the abdominal muscles flat, and the shoulders relaxed.

Avoid lifting your back too high—this forces the spine out of alignment and puts stress on the neck and upper back.

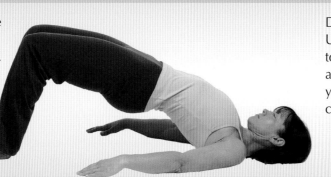

Don't arch your back. Use your abdominals to lift your hips into alignment with your knees and chest.

Gentle rotation is great for releasing tension from the middle of your back and stretching your waist and the sides of your body. Rotation exercises for the spine also help to lengthen the waist and stretch and strengthen the oblique muscles that are used to twist the body. This reduces pressure on the spine and helps to streamline your shape.

Correct practice

Before you begin, make sure your head, neck, and shoulders are relaxed on the floor. Place a pillow under your head if you need to relieve tension in this area.

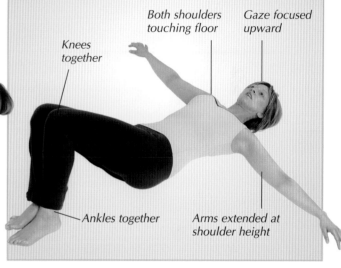

Knees together

Both shoulders touching floor

Gaze focused upward

Ankles together

Arms extended at shoulder height

1 Lie on your back in neutral with your knees bent and feet flat on the floor. Keep your knees and ankles together as if they were one leg and spread your arms to the sides at about shoulder height. **Inhale** to prepare.

2 As you exhale, contract your abdominal muscles and slowly sway your knees and hips to the right as far as you can, keeping your left shoulder on the floor. Keep your knees and ankles together and the outer edge of your left foot on the floor. **Inhale** while your knees are rotated.

3 As you exhale, bring your knees back into neutral. Keep your gaze focused upward to the ceiling. **Inhale** while in neutral.

4 As you exhale, smoothly sway your knees to the left, checking that your right shoulder is imprinting into the floor. **Inhale** while your knees are rotated.

5 As you exhale, bring your knees back into neutral. Keep your gaze focused upward to the ceiling.

Repeat 4–6 times in a slow, flowing movement.

The Single-Leg Knee Floating exercise works the muscles around the pelvis, abdomen, buttocks, lower back, and hips. Strengthening these muscles improves pelvic stability and helps correct lower-back problems.

Although this looks like a simple exercise, it is extremely effective for keeping the hip joints mobile, strong, and healthy. It also reduces the risk of osteoporosis in later life.

Pelvic alignment

To make sure your pelvis stays in neutral while doing this exercise, focus on your abdominal muscles and move only from the hip joints. Use the sacrum and tailbone as a gauge for keeping the pelvis in neutral—with the tailbone extending and the sacrum imprinting into the floor.

You may want to place your hands on your pelvis with fingertips on your pubic bone and heels of your hands on your hipbones to feel that your pelvis is remaining still and in alignment while your legs are moving.

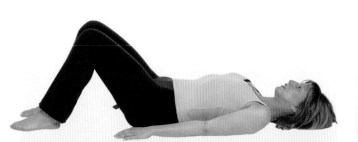

1 Lie on your back in neutral with your knees bent and feet flat on the floor. Check that your ankles, knees, and hips are in alignment and your ankles and knees are hip-distance apart. **Inhale** to prepare.

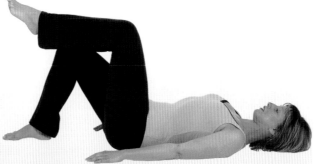

2 As you exhale, use your hip flexor muscles to slowly float your left leg up until the knee is directly over the hip and the ankle and knee form a horizontal line. **Inhale** in this position.

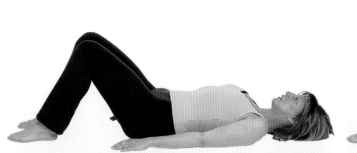

3 As you exhale, draw down through the ribs, pull in the abdominal muscles tightly, and float your left foot gently back down to the floor.
Inhale to prepare for working with your right leg.

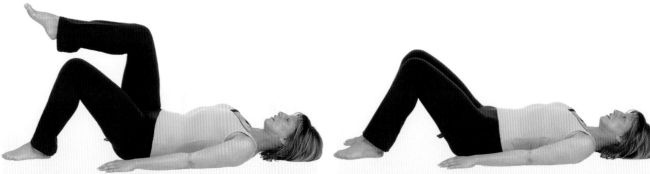

4 As you exhale, float your right leg up to the right-angle position. Make sure that your knee is aligned over the hip.
Inhale slowly in this position.

5 As you exhale, gently float your leg back down.

Repeat 6 times in a smooth, continuous movement.

In this exercise you move only your legs while the rest of your body, including your hip joints, stays still and relaxed. As you slide your legs in and out, your pelvis is stabilized by your abdominal muscles, which keep you in a neutral spine position. Practicing this improves pelvic stability and encourages economy of movement.

Leg Slides require great control of the core muscles of the torso and are excellent for flattening your tummy muscles.

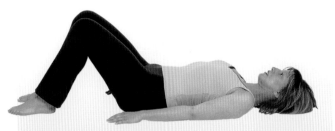

1 Lie on your back in neutral with your knees bent and hip-distance apart, arms by your sides, and feet parallel and flat on the floor.

Adding a flex and point

You can add a flex and point of the foot to this exercise between steps 2 and 3.

Flexing and pointing the feet on the exhale and inhale helps you to feel the muscles of your legs lengthen and engage, especially the calf muscles. This gives your calf muscles a gentle stretch and in turn engages the muscles of the legs to assist in the stability of the pelvis.

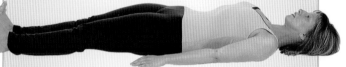

In the stretch position, flex your feet **as you exhale.**

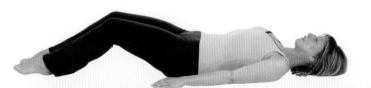

2 **As you inhale,** gently slide your legs along the floor to a straight position, keeping your heels lightly in

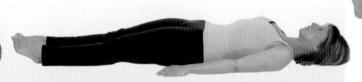

contact with the floor. During the slide, keep your pelvis in neutral and your shoulders relaxed.

As you inhale, point your feet. Then, **as you exhale,** slide your heels back in.

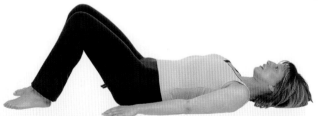

3 **As you exhale,** contract down through the ribs, engage your abdominal muscles, draw the pelvic floor muscles in toward your center, and imprint the sacrum into the floor to retain neutral pelvis. Smoothly draw your legs back toward the buttocks into knees-bent position. As you draw in your legs, drag your

heels lightly along the floor as if you are trying to create grooves in it. Keep your shoulders and arms relaxed.

Repeat 4–6 times in a flowing movement.

Pelvic alignment

Remember to stabilize your pelvis with your abdominal muscles while slowly sliding your legs up and down. Your pelvis should stay in its neutral position throughout the exercise.

Most of us spend too many hours sitting hunched over a desk, a book, or a computer! As a result, we carry a lot of unnecessary tension through the shoulder, chest, and neck areas. The Ribcage Arms exercise helps to relieve tension in the upper back, shoulders, and neck. It gently stretches the latissimus dorsi muscles in your back and strengthens the muscles around the shoulder blades, improving the range of motion in the shoulder joints.

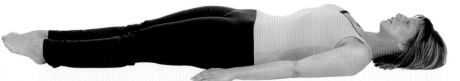

1 Lie on your back in neutral with your legs fully extended, feet hip-distance apart, arms by your sides, neck and shoulders relaxed, and the shoulder blades imprinting into the floor. Focus your gaze toward the ceiling.

4 As you inhale, slowly and smoothly float up your arms until your fingertips are pointing to the ceiling again.

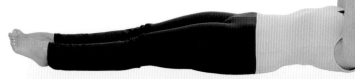

2 As you inhale, slowly float your arms toward the ceiling until your fingertips are pointing straight up. As your arms move, keep your shoulders relaxed and imprinting down into the floor.

5 As you exhale, gently float your arms back down to the floor by your sides.

Repeat 4–6 times in a smooth, continuous movement.

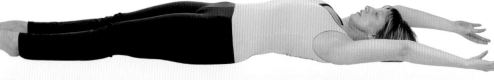

3 As you exhale, soften down through the breastbone, contract the abdominal muscles, and move your arms behind your head as far as your shoulders allow. Don't let your lumbar spine lift as you extend your arms—work within the range your shoulder flexibility will allow.

With knees bent

If you have tight muscles in your lower back or lordosis (arched lower back), you can do Ribcage Arms with your knees bent and feet flat on the floor. This will help to prevent moving the spine out of neutral when you extend your arms over your head.

Here you combine Leg Slides with Ribcage Arms in a coordinated and controlled movement. Your legs and arms should work together. Make sure that they move at the same speed so that they complete each movement at the same time. This exercise emphasizes control of the hip flexors and shoulder joints while the core muscles stabilize the body.

Correct practice

It is important to practice this exercise slowly so you can focus on controlling your breathing and your leg and arm movements while keeping your pelvis in neutral. Make sure your arms move at the same speed as your legs.

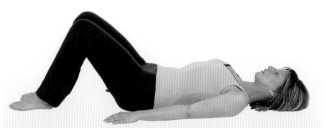

1 Lie on your back in neutral with your knees bent and hip-distance apart and arms relaxed at your sides.

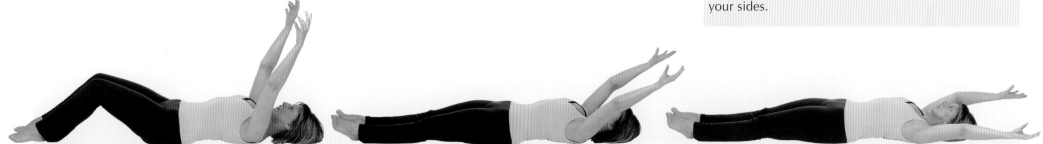

2 As you inhale, gently slide your legs along the floor and, at the same time, slowly float your arms up and over your head. As you slide your legs, keep the heels lightly in contact with the floor. Use your abdominal muscles to keep your pelvis in neutral, with your tailbone extended, sacrum pressing down, and lower spine retaining its natural curve. Touch your arms to the floor if possible, but don't arch your back. Keep your shoulders relaxed and imprinting into the floor.

3 As you exhale, return to the neutral spine position by bringing your arms up and back down to your sides. At the same time, slide your legs back up while contracting through the pelvic floor and abdominal muscles, softening through the ribs, and stabilizing the pelvis in neutral.

Repeat 4–6 times in a flowing movement.

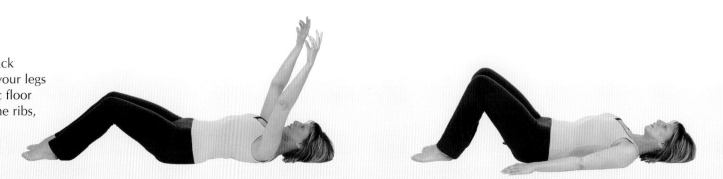

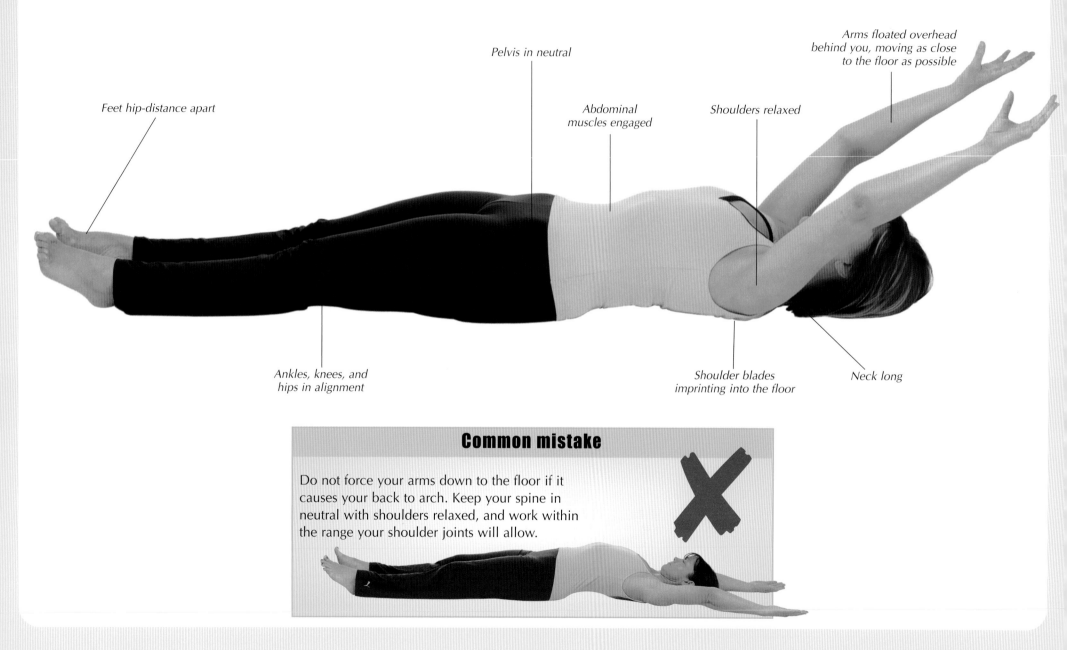

Pelvis in neutral

Arms floated overhead behind you, moving as close to the floor as possible

Feet hip-distance apart

Abdominal muscles engaged

Shoulders relaxed

Ankles, knees, and hips in alignment

Shoulder blades imprinting into the floor

Neck long

Common mistake

Do not force your arms down to the floor if it causes your back to arch. Keep your spine in neutral with shoulders relaxed, and work within the range your shoulder joints will allow.

SINGLE ARM SLIDES

Like Ribcage Arms, the Single Arm Slides exercise mobilizes your shoulder joints, relieving stiffness in the upper back and shoulder area. At the same time, because of the addition of a pelvic tilt, this exercise lengthens the erector muscles of the back. Especially good for people with rounded shoulders (kyphosis), this exercise helps to open the front of the chest by gently stretching the pectoral muscles.

1 Lie with your knees bent and hip-distance apart, pelvis in neutral, and shoulders relaxed. Place your arms on the floor with your elbows in a right-angle position and the back of the forearms and the hands touching the floor. **Inhale** slowly to prepare.

2 **As you exhale,** engage the abdominal muscles, draw the pelvic floor muscles in, and bring your pelvis up so that your pubic bone tilts toward your navel. As you do this, gently extend your right arm behind your head as far as you can, keeping your elbow on the floor as you slide your arm.

3 **As you inhale,** return your pelvis to neutral and slowly draw your arm back down to the right-angle position.

4 **As you exhale,** tilt your pelvis as before. As you do this, extend your left arm.
As you inhale, return your pelvis to neutral and your arm to the right-angle position.

Repeat 4–6 times in a flowing movement.

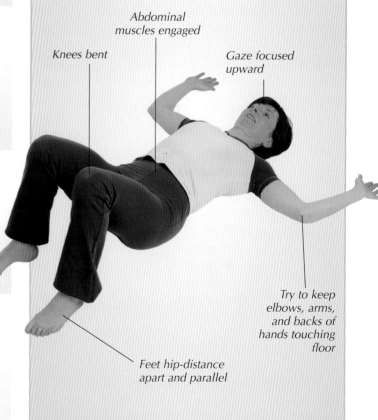

Correct practice

If your shoulders and chest muscles are tight, you may find it hard to keep your elbows on the floor when sliding your arms. Do not force them down. At first, rest the backs of your hands on the floor as you exercise and gradually, with practice, your elbows will sink nearer to the floor as your shoulder and chest muscles lengthen and relax. If you experience any sharp pains, do not continue.

Abdominal muscles engaged

Knees bent

Gaze focused upward

Try to keep elbows, arms, and backs of hands touching floor

Feet hip-distance apart and parallel

You use your hamstrings when you flex and bend your knees or stretch your thighs. These tendons also help to hold the pelvis in place and keep your lower spine mobile. Your hamstrings become shortened by poor posture when sitting or standing. They also get shorter during exercise, so always stretch them afterward to return them to their normal length.

Tight hamstrings pull your pelvis out of alignment and flatten the lumbar spine, which reduces flexibility. To test whether yours are tight, sit on the floor with your legs stretched out. If you can sit upright with your hips over your sitz bones, you have healthy, flexible hamstrings—if not, your hamstrings are tight.

Common mistake

Holding your leg with your hands while stretching your hamstrings can force your shoulders to lift off the floor and your head to tilt back as shown here. Prevent this by using a towel or belt for this exercise. Keep your elbows on the floor beside you and focus on keeping your pelvic alignment in neutral.

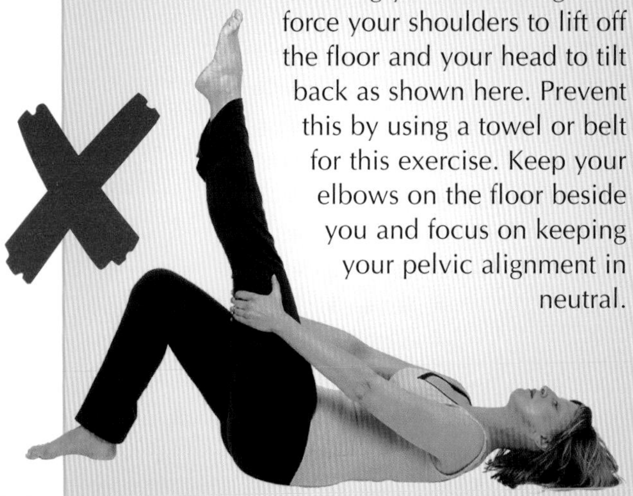

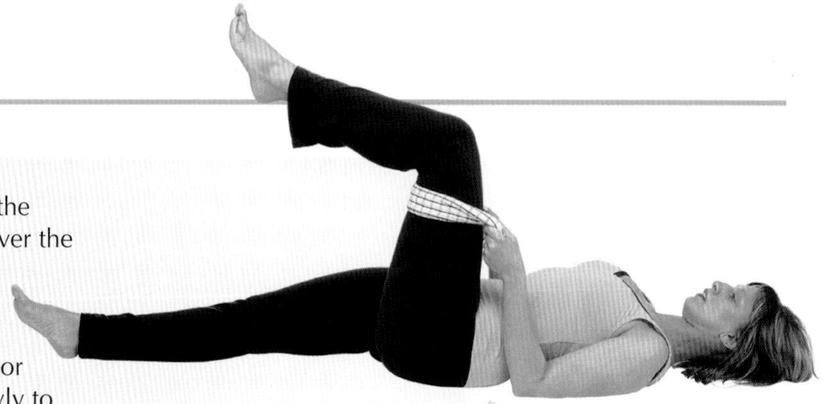

1 Lie on your back. Float your left leg up into the right-angle position, with the knee directly over the hips and the ankle and knee aligned to form a near horizontal line. Place a small towel, cloth, or belt around your thigh and hold one end in each hand. Keep your elbows on the floor so that your shoulders stay relaxed. **Inhale** slowly to prepare for the stretching.

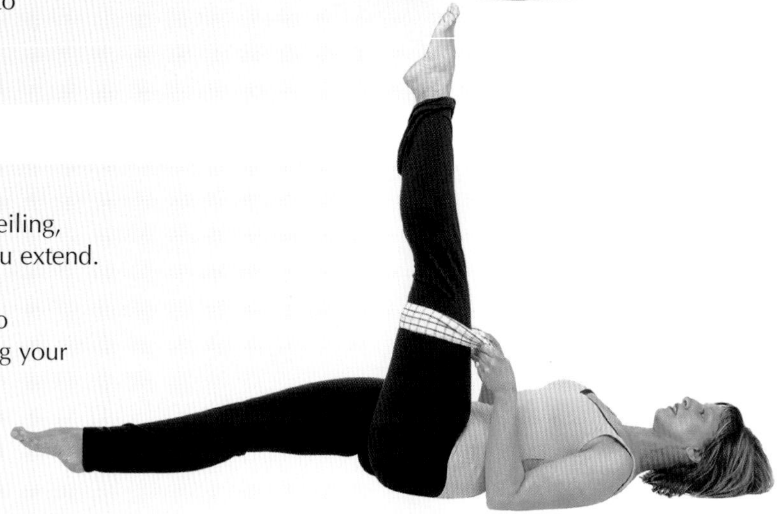

2 **As you exhale,** extend your left leg toward the ceiling, keeping your knee directly above your hip as you extend. **As you inhale,** breathe deeply into your back. **As you exhale,** stretch the right leg along the floor to lengthen through the hip flexors. Focus on extending your left leg upward while holding the pelvis in neutral, rather than pulling the leg toward you. Hold this position for a few breaths, just breathing deeply in through the nose and out through the mouth while allowing the hamstrings to stretch.

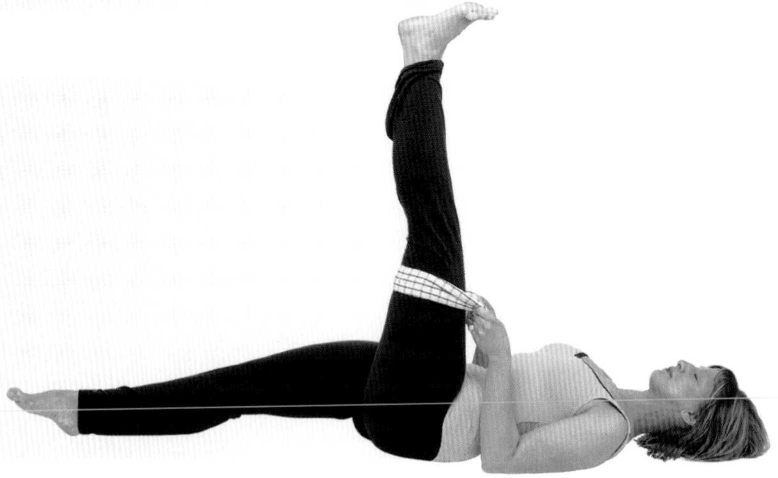

3 While the left leg is still stretching, point the foot **as you inhale.** **As you exhale,** flex the foot. This flexing increases the stretch on the calf muscles. **As you inhale,** release the left leg down.

Repeat with the right leg.

Having mastered the exercises in this chapter, link them together in this flowing 10–12-minute routine. Only abbreviated instructions are given here. If you need reminders of the precise movements, refer back to the pages indicated.

As you repeat each exercise and as you move from one exercise to the next, keep the movements flowing smoothly in time with your slow, deep, ribcage breathing. If you need to rest, practice your ribcage breathing while lying in neutral, before starting the next exercise.

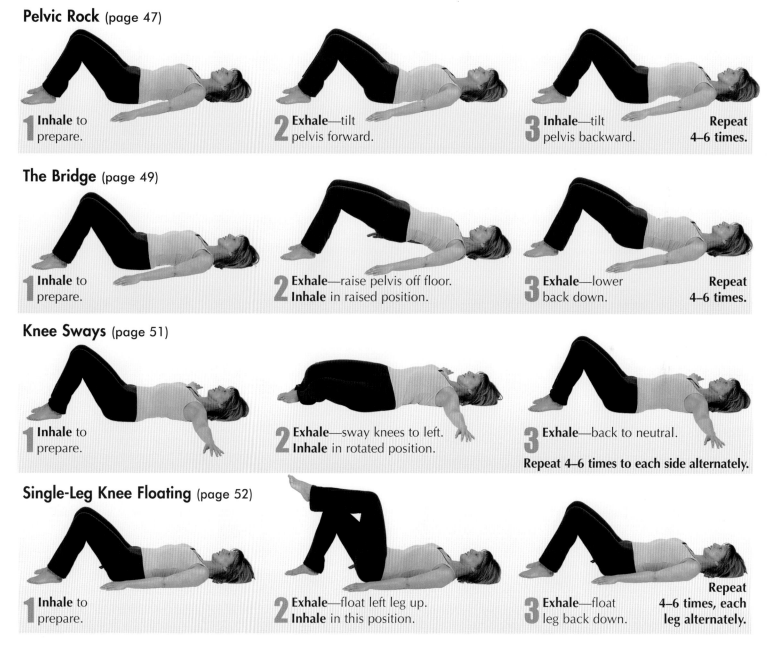

Pelvic Rock (page 47)

1 Inhale to prepare.

2 Exhale—tilt pelvis forward.

3 Inhale—tilt pelvis backward.   **Repeat 4–6 times.**

The Bridge (page 49)

1 Inhale to prepare.

2 Exhale—raise pelvis off floor. Inhale in raised position.

3 Exhale—lower back down.   **Repeat 4–6 times.**

Knee Sways (page 51)

1 Inhale to prepare.

2 Exhale—sway knees to left. Inhale in rotated position.

3 Exhale—back to neutral.

Repeat 4–6 times to each side alternately.

Single-Leg Knee Floating (page 52)

1 Inhale to prepare.

2 Exhale—float left leg up. Inhale in this position.

3 Exhale—float leg back down.   **Repeat 4–6 times, each leg alternately.**

continued on next page

Leg Slides with Ribcage Arms (page 55)

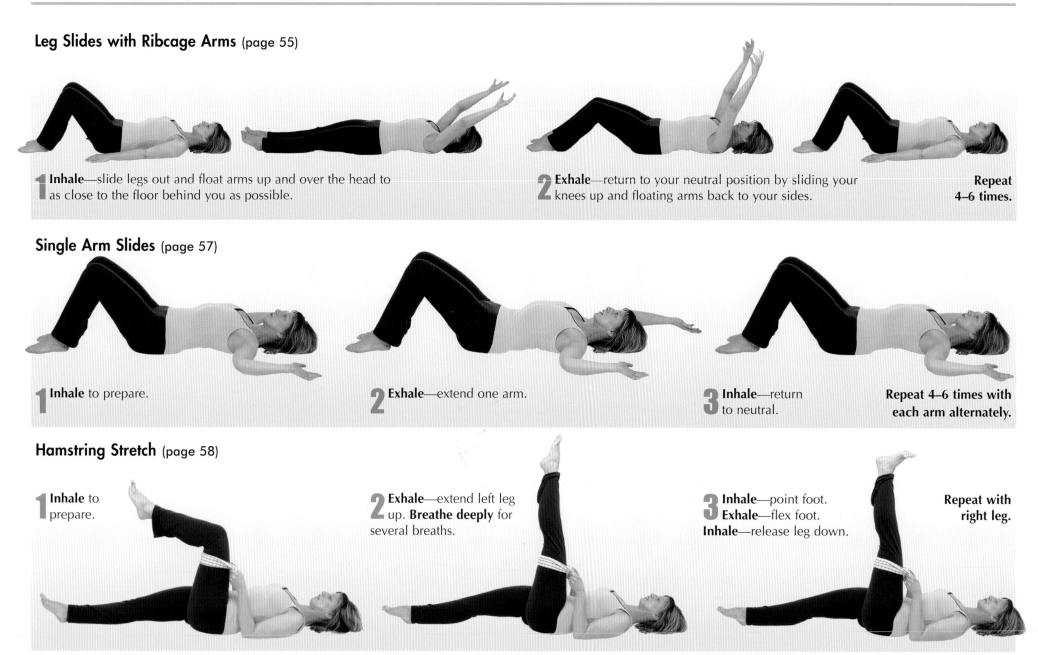

1 Inhale—slide legs out and float arms up and over the head to as close to the floor behind you as possible.

2 Exhale—return to your neutral position by sliding your knees up and floating arms back to your sides.

Repeat 4–6 times.

Single Arm Slides (page 57)

1 Inhale to prepare.

2 Exhale—extend one arm.

3 Inhale—return to neutral.

Repeat 4–6 times with each arm alternately.

Hamstring Stretch (page 58)

1 Inhale to prepare.

2 Exhale—extend left leg up. **Breathe deeply** for several breaths.

3 Inhale—point foot. Exhale—flex foot. Inhale—release leg down.

Repeat with right leg.

6

Back Lengthening and Strengthening

About back lengthening and strengthening

Practicing these exercises will improve your shoulder alignment for good posture and increase the flexibility of your spine.

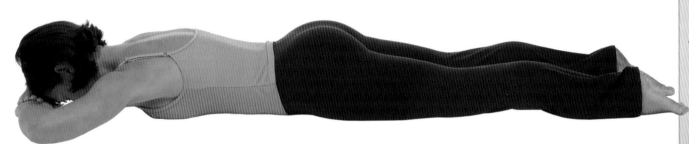

Lying on your front in neutral

- Rest your forehead on your hands. Draw your chin in, focus your gaze toward the floor, and extend the top of your head away from your torso.

- Draw your shoulders away from your neck. Relax the back of your ribcage and shoulders.

- Keep your pubic bone and hipbones in alignment and imprinting into the floor. Engage your pelvic floor and abdominal muscles to prevent the lumbar curve from over-exaggerating. Extend your tailbone away from your torso.

- Lengthen through your legs, keeping the ankles, knees, and hips in alignment.

The muscles of the back and front of your torso work together to stabilize your body, keeping your bones and muscles in balance. The oblique and transversus muscles wrap around your torso and are attached to the back of the ribcage and the spine. So when you are exercising on your stomach, you are working both your back muscles and abdominal muscles. Working your back muscles while lying on your front will give you a more defined shape, especially around the bra line. It will also strengthen the erector muscles, muscles that run along the spine, which will improve your shoulder alignment and make your back more flexible.

Before beginning the exercises, review your neutral spine position (see top right) and practice your rhythmic deep breathing.

CAUTION: Do not lie on your stomach if you are over 12 weeks pregnant.

Breathing practice

- **As you inhale**, expand your ribcage sideways and backward toward the ceiling.

- **As you exhale**, pull your navel in toward your spine, close the front of your ribcage and draw up through your pelvic floor muscles. Imprint the triangle of your pubic bone and hipbones into the floor, creating a small cavity under your belly.

- Keep your shoulders and neck relaxed and your pelvis in neutral while breathing.

The muscles of your back play an integral part in maintaining good posture. We all tend to spend a lot of our time sitting with our abdominal and back muscles disengaged. So these muscles become weak and create unbalanced posture. This exercise will help to mobilize and lengthen the lumbar spine as well as improve abdominal strength.

When performing the Pelvic Tilt, you may want to place a thin cushion under your pelvis for more comfort.

On the exhale...

- Make sure your pubic bone and hipbones create a tripod as the navel draws in and up on the exhale.

- Try to lift the navel off the floor and toward the spine, creating a space under the belly.

- Engage your pelvic floor and abdominal muscles to prevent the lower back from over-exaggerating the concave lumbar curve.

- Lengthen through the legs, keeping the ankles, knees, and hips in alignment.

1 Lie on your front in neutral with your forehead resting on the back of your hands, your elbows bent, and your legs hip-distance apart and lengthening along the floor. **Inhale** slowly and deeply through your nose, breathing into the back of your ribcage.

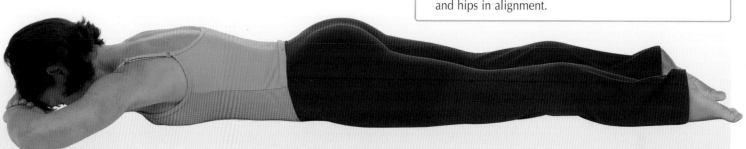

2 **As you exhale,** slowly tilt your pelvis toward your navel so that your pubic bone imprints into the floor and you can feel your lumbar spine lengthen. Make sure your abdominals are pulling in toward the spine and the front of the ribcage is closed to engage the transversus muscle that supports the torso. Keep your shoulders and upper back relaxed and your legs lengthened. **As you inhale,** release back to neutral.

Repeat 4–6 times.

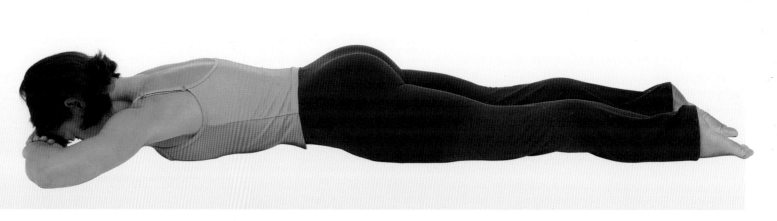

With practice, the Single Leg Lift will improve your ability to keep your spine in neutral while you lift your leg from the hip joint. To gain this control, the exercise uses the gluteus muscles (the buttocks), so it will also help to streamline your bottom, hips, and thighs and strengthen your lower back.

Correct practice

- Balance on the triangle formed by your pubic bone and two hipbones as your navel draws off the floor.

- Keep your pelvis in neutral as you lift your leg so that your lower back does not curve inward too much.

- Relax the front of your ribcage as you lift your leg to help engage the transversus muscle.

- Keep your upper back, shoulders, and neck relaxed.

1 Lie on your front in neutral with your forehead resting on the back of your hands, your elbows bent, and your legs hip-distance apart and lengthening along the floor. Make sure your pubic bone and both hipbones are in contact with the floor. **Inhale** slowly and deeply through your nose, broadening through your back, to prepare.

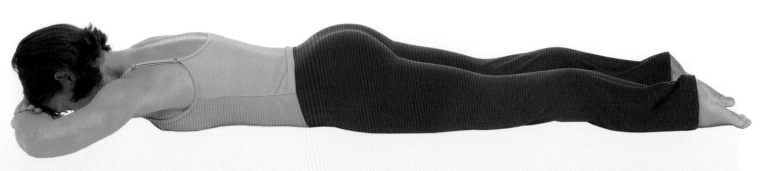

2 **As you exhale,** pull your navel off the floor toward your spine and at the same time, slowly lengthen and lift your left leg, keeping both hipbones on the floor. Extend the tailbone to keep your pelvis in neutral. **As you inhale,** slowly and gently lower your leg back to the floor.

Repeat 4–6 times, alternating legs.

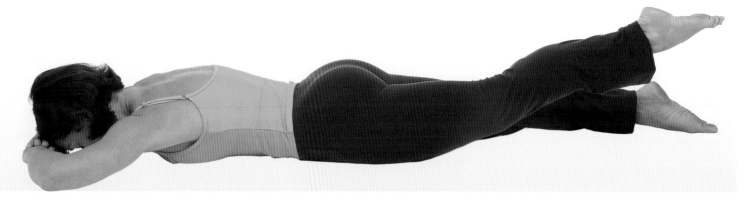

Floating your chest off the floor works the muscles of the back and helps to keep a healthy balance between your abdominal muscles and your back muscles. Most forms of exercise tend to focus more on the front of the body, leaving the back muscles undeveloped, which encourages bad posture. Chest Floating will improve the strength of your back and shoulder area. It is especially good for people who have a sedentary job and for those with rounded shoulders.

Correct practice

- The body cannot bend back as far as it can bend forward, so do not expect as great a range of movement when performing exercises lying prone.

- Think about lengthening the chest forward as you lift to keep the stabilizing muscles engaged.

1 Lie on your front in neutral with your arms extending along the sides of your body and the tip of your nose on the floor. Keep your pelvis in neutral and your legs extending along the floor. **Inhale** slowly to prepare, and check that your shoulders are relaxed and down.

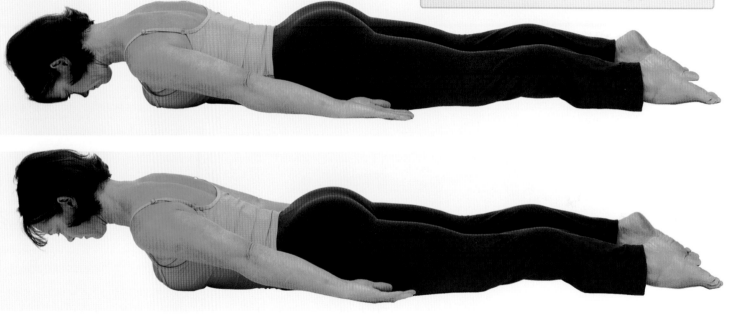

2 **As you exhale,** draw your abdominals in, lengthen your arms along the sides of your body, draw your shoulders away from your ears, and slowly float your head, neck, and chest off the floor. Engage your pelvic floor muscles to maintain neutral pelvis.

3 **As you inhale,** lower your head, neck, and chest back down, drawing the shoulders away from the neck and lengthening your arms along your sides to help keep your shoulders stable.

Repeat 4–6 times in a smooth, continuous movement.

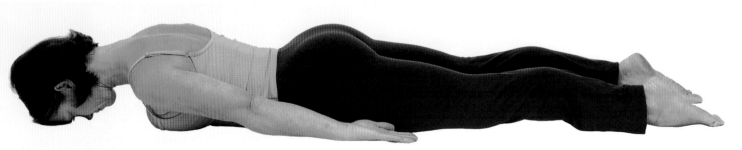

Lateral rotation added to Chest Floating strengthens the oblique muscles around the waist and the latissimus dorsi (one of the major muscles of the back). Practicing this exercise will gradually increase your range of movement.

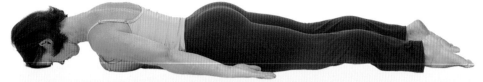

1 Lie on your front in neutral with your arms extending along your sides and the tip of your nose on the floor. Keep your pelvis in neutral and your legs extending. **Inhale** slowly to prepare, and check that your shoulders are relaxed and down.

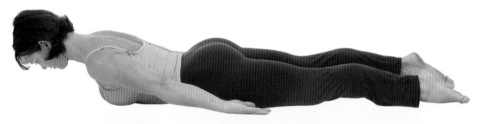

2 **As you exhale,** draw your abdominals in while lengthening your arms, drawing your shoulders away from your ears, and slowly floating your head, neck, and chest off the floor. Engage your pelvic floor muscles to maintain neutral pelvis. **Inhale** slowly while holding this elevated position.

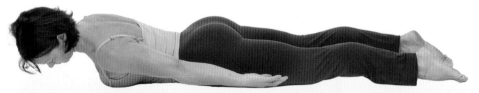

3 **As you exhale,** slowly tilt your body to the left, bringing your left shoulder closer to your left hip. (The movement is similar to a standing side bend.)

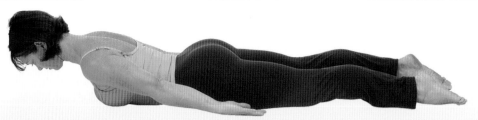

4 **As you inhale,** slowly bring your shoulders back into alignment at the center.

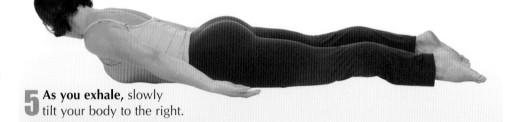

5 **As you exhale,** slowly tilt your body to the right.

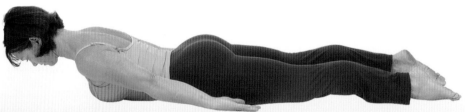

6 **As you inhale,** slowly bring your shoulders back into alignment at the center.

7 **As you exhale,** slowly lower your chest, head, and neck back to the floor.

Repeat 4–6 times in a flowing, continuous movement.

This exercise challenges the muscles responsible for your core stability when you lift one arm and leg off the floor while trying to maintain your neutral spine position. It also lengthens the hip flexor muscles that run from the front of the knee to the hip.

1 Lie on your front in neutral with your arms straight and extending forward and the tip of your nose on the floor. Keep your pelvis in neutral and your legs extending along the floor. **Inhale** slowly to prepare.

2 **As you exhale,** draw your abdominals in and engage your pelvic floor muscles to maintain neutral and prevent the lower back from curving inward too much. Slowly raise your right leg and left arm off the floor. Lengthen through the arm and leg as you lift. Keep your left shoulder stable and not hunched toward your head.

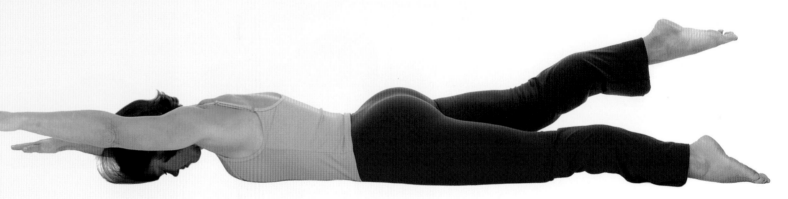

3 **As you inhale,** lower your arm and leg back to the floor.

Repeat 4–6 times, alternating left arm and right leg with right arm and left leg.

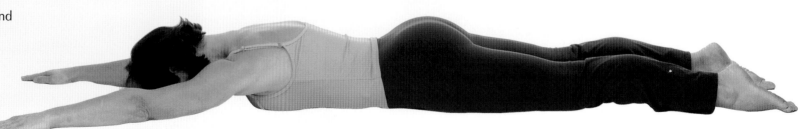

SWIMMING

The aim of this exercise is to increase the range of your shoulder movement by strengthening the muscles of the upper back. For the exercise to be effective, be sure to keep your upper back, shoulders, and neck relaxed.

1 Lie on your front in neutral with your arms straight and extending forward and the tip of your nose on the floor. Keep your pelvis in neutral and your legs extending along the floor. **Inhale** slowly to prepare.

2 **As you exhale,** pull your abdominal muscles in, lengthen through the legs (but keep them on the floor), draw your shoulders down your back, and lift your head, neck, and chest off the floor, sweeping your arms around to your sides.

3 **As you inhale,** slowly sweep your arms back to the forward position and, at the same time, lower your head, neck, and chest back to the floor.

Repeat 4–6 times.

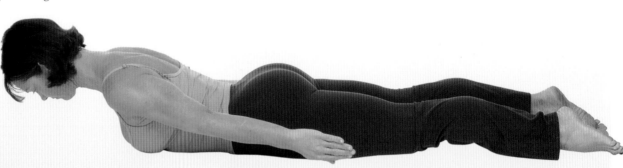

Correct practice

- Remember your triangle! When lying in the neutral spine position, your pubic bone and two hipbones form a triangle on the floor. Balance on these three bones as your navel draws off the floor.

- Keep your pelvis in neutral as you lift your upper body so that your lower back does not curve inward too much.

- Extend the top of your head forward as you lift your upper body, keeping the neck vertebrae in line with the upper spine.

The Swan is another valuable exercise for strengthening the upper back muscles while stabilizing the torso. It also improves the range of movement in your upper back.

1 Lie on your front in neutral with the tip of your nose on the floor and your arms at a right angle, palms on the floor. Keep your pelvis in neutral and your legs hip-distance apart and extending along the floor. **Inhale** to prepare.

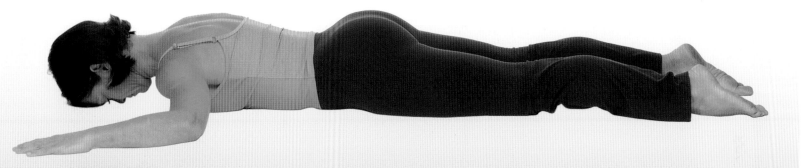

2 As you exhale, draw your abdominals in, draw your shoulders away from your ears, and slowly float your head, neck, and chest off the floor. Extend your breastbone forward as you lift, keeping your elbows on the floor. Engage your pelvic floor muscles to maintain neutral pelvis.

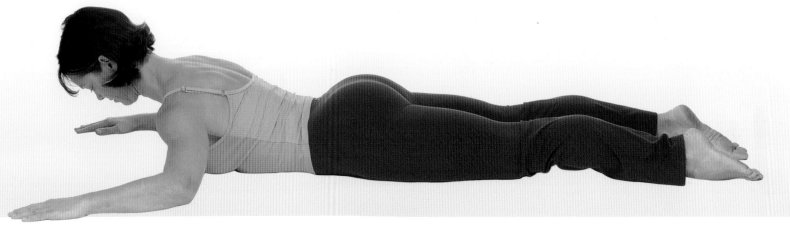

3 As you inhale, slowly lower your chest back down to the floor.

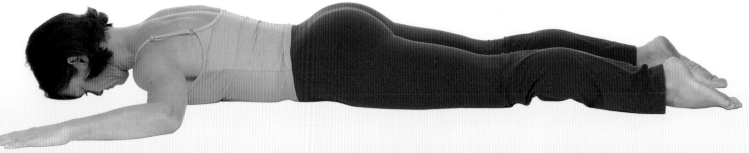

Repeat 4–6 times in a slow, flowing movement.

This stretch is widely used in many fitness regimes. It is extremely beneficial if you have tight hip flexor and quadriceps muscles. Knee problems are sometimes caused by tight quadriceps muscles, so practicing this exercise regularly can help to alleviate the problem.

Have a small towel or scarf near you to assist with the stretch.

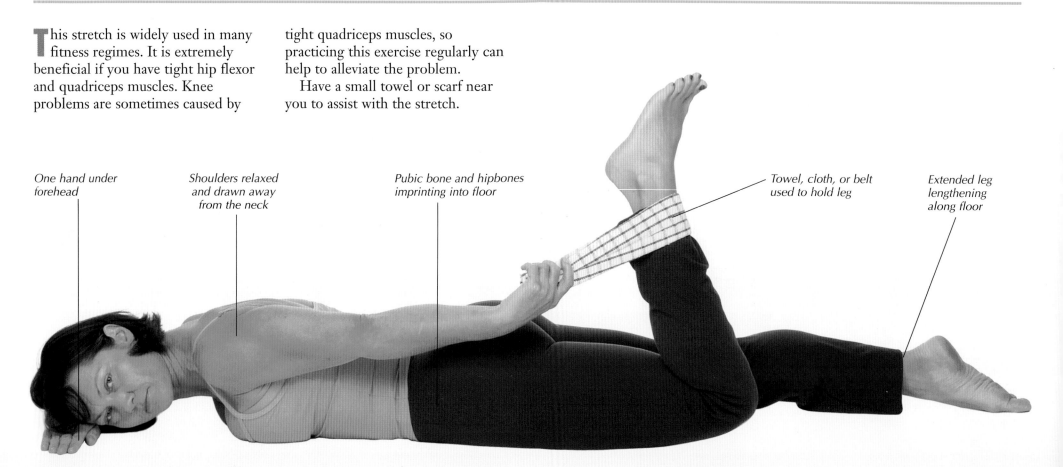

One hand under forehead

Shoulders relaxed and drawn away from the neck

Pubic bone and hipbones imprinting into floor

Towel, cloth, or belt used to hold leg

Extended leg lengthening along floor

Lie on your front and bend your left knee. Wrap a towel or scarf around your left ankle or lower leg and hold the ends in your left hand. Put your right hand under your forehead with your head facing to the left or toward the floor. Check that your knees are together and your right leg is lengthening along the floor. Your pubic bone and hipbones should be imprinting into the floor and your tailbone lengthening toward your heels. Relax your chest into the floor, drawing relaxed shoulders away from the neck.

Inhale into your upper back, expanding the ribcage.
As you exhale, pull your abdominal muscles in toward the spine, creating a cavity under your navel. Tilt your pelvis toward your navel to imprint your pubic bone and hipbones into the floor.
Inhale in the stretched position.
As you exhale, deepen the pelvic tilt to increase the stretch.
Inhale and release.

Repeat with the right leg.

This 10–12-minute routine is made up of the exercises you have learned in this chapter. Use it if you want to focus on improving your back flexibility or your shoulder alignment.

Lie on your front in neutral and do some deep breathing before starting. Then follow the routine in the sequence given, keeping the movements flowing together in time with your rhythmic ribcage breathing.

CAUTION: Do not lie on your stomach if you are over 12 weeks pregnant.

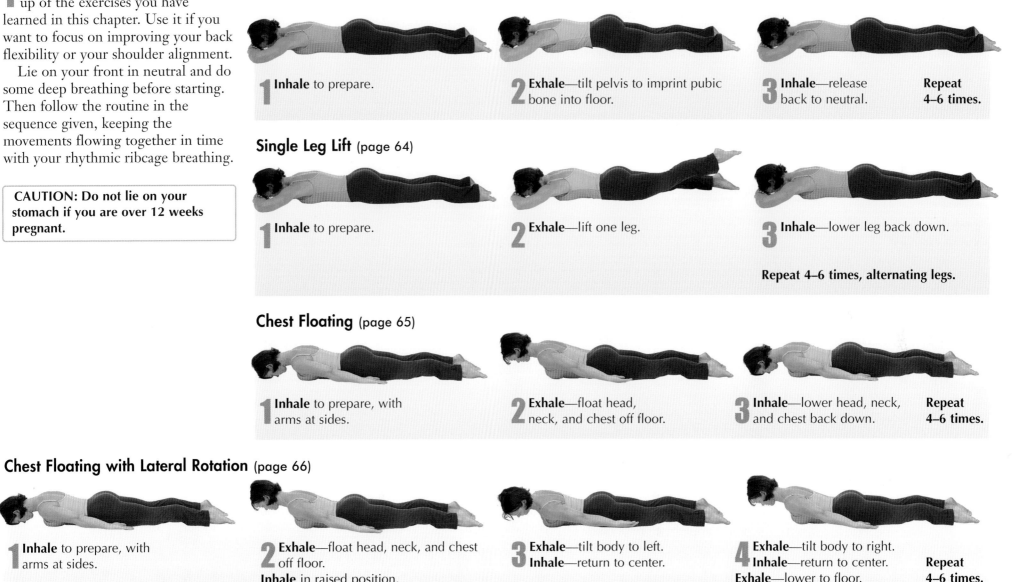

Pelvic Tilt (page 63)

1 **Inhale** to prepare.

2 **Exhale**—tilt pelvis to imprint pubic bone into floor.

3 **Inhale**—release back to neutral.

Repeat 4–6 times.

Single Leg Lift (page 64)

1 **Inhale** to prepare.

2 **Exhale**—lift one leg.

3 **Inhale**—lower leg back down.

Repeat 4–6 times, alternating legs.

Chest Floating (page 65)

1 **Inhale** to prepare, with arms at sides.

2 **Exhale**—float head, neck, and chest off floor.

3 **Inhale**—lower head, neck, and chest back down.

Repeat 4–6 times.

Chest Floating with Lateral Rotation (page 66)

1 **Inhale** to prepare, with arms at sides.

2 **Exhale**—float head, neck, and chest off floor.
Inhale in raised position.

3 **Exhale**—tilt body to left.
Inhale—return to center.

4 **Exhale**—tilt body to right.
Inhale—return to center.
Exhale—lower to floor.

Repeat 4–6 times.

continued on next page

Opposite Arm and Leg Raise (page 67)

1 **Inhale** to prepare, with arms extended.

2 **Exhale**—raise right leg and left arm, keeping the body relaxed and in neutral.

3 **Inhale**—lower back down.

Repeat 4–6 times, alternating left arm and right leg with right arm and left leg.

Swimming (page 68)

1 **Inhale** to prepare, with arms extended.

2 **Exhale**—lift head, neck, and chest, and sweep arms to sides.

3 **Inhale**—lower back down and sweep arms forward.

Repeat 4–6 times.

The Swan (page 69)

1 **Inhale** to prepare, with arms at right angles.

2 **Exhale**—float head, neck, and chest off floor.

3 **Inhale**—lower back down.

Repeat 4–6 times.

Quad and Hip Flexor Stretch
(page 70)

Wrap towel around left leg and hold with hand. **Inhale** to prepare.
Exhale—tilt pelvis to imprint pubic bone and hipbones into floor.
Inhale in stretched position.
Exhale—deepen tilt. **Inhale**—release.

Repeat with right leg.

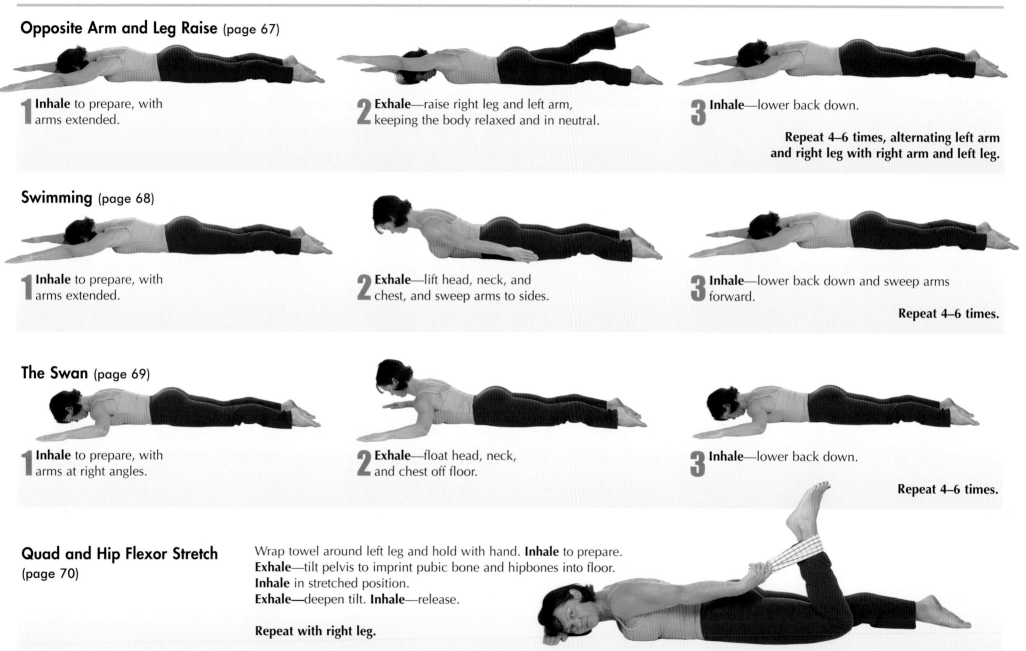

7 Staying Strong

About exercising on all fours

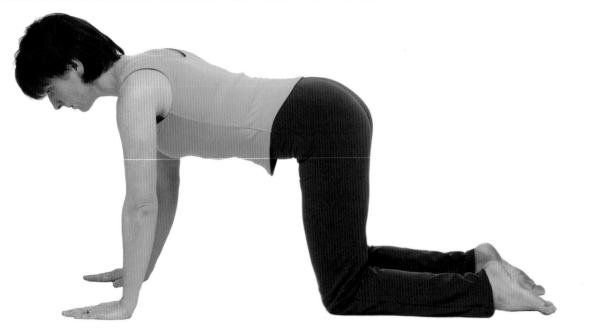

Exercises done kneeling on all fours are designed to improve the mobility and flexibility of your spine. They will strengthen the abdominal and back muscles and generally improve your posture.

Take the time to get into the correct neutral position and to practice your breathing (see right) before starting these exercises.

Working in a kneeling position on all fours may make your knees feel a bit uncomfortable. If so, give yourself more padding—place a thin cushion under your knees for extra comfort. If your wrists feel stiff or uncomfortable when your palms are flat on the floor, try placing a soft, foam, tennis-size ball under each hand to raise your palms and relieve pressure on the wrists.

On all fours in neutral

- Kneel on all fours and maintain neutral spine. Position your arms shoulder-width apart, palms down, and fingers facing forward.

- Line up your wrists and elbows directly under your shoulders. Draw your shoulders down the back, away from your neck. Lengthen your neck and extend the top of your head forward.

- Position your knees hip-distance apart and directly underneath your hips. Extend your tailbone and engage your pelvic floor muscles.

- Engage your abdominal muscles to hold your torso in neutral and prevent the lumbar curve from over-exaggerating. To resist gravity, focus on drawing your navel inward and upward.

- When doing the exercises, keep your elbow joints soft and your shoulders back and down.

Breathing practice

When correctly positioned, practice ribcage breathing.

- **As you inhale,** expand your ribcage sideways and backward.

- **As you exhale,** engage your pelvic floor muscles to draw your navel inward and upward and close the front of the ribcage without moving your spine or pelvis.

The aim of this stretch is to improve flexibility of the spine, lengthen the back muscles, and improve awareness of correct breathing, neutral spine, and abdominal stability. It is a good exercise to practice when your back is aching (or if you are pregnant, when your back feels uncomfortable). It is also a good alternative to exercising the abdominal muscles when lying on your back.

Although the Cat Stretch can be difficult to master at first, using visualization will help you to move your spine correctly. Imagine that your vertebrae are a string of pearls and that you are moving each one individually, one at a time, as you move your spine upward and downward, into and out of the arched position.

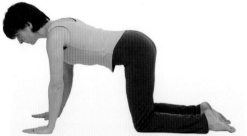 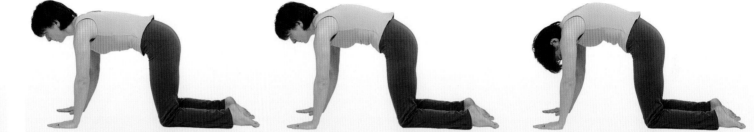

1 Kneel on all fours in neutral and check your alignment. **Inhale** to prepare.

2 **As you exhale,** slowly and smoothly arch your spine, starting at the tailbone end. Point the tailbone down toward the floor by tilting the pelvis, then sequentially round the lower back, the middle back, through the shoulder blades, and down through the neck so that your head lengthens toward the floor and your back arches like an angry cat.
Inhale slowly in this arched position, expanding the back and the shoulders.

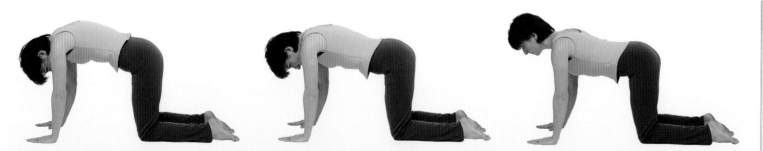 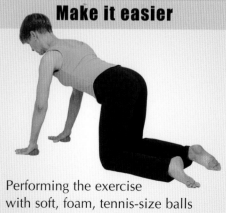

Make it easier

3 **As you exhale,** gently move your spine back into neutral, starting at the tailbone end. Extend the tailbone back to bring the pelvis into neutral, followed by the lower back, the middle back, then between the shoulder blades, through the neck, and extend the top of the head forward. Make sure that the abdominal and pelvic floor muscles are engaged as you come back into the neutral spine position.

Repeat 4–6 times in a slow, continuous movement.

Performing the exercise with soft, foam, tennis-size balls under your palms can relieve any discomfort in the wrists.

CAT STRETCH IN FOCUS

Correct practice
Move into and out of the arched position starting at the tailbone and moving each vertebra individually.

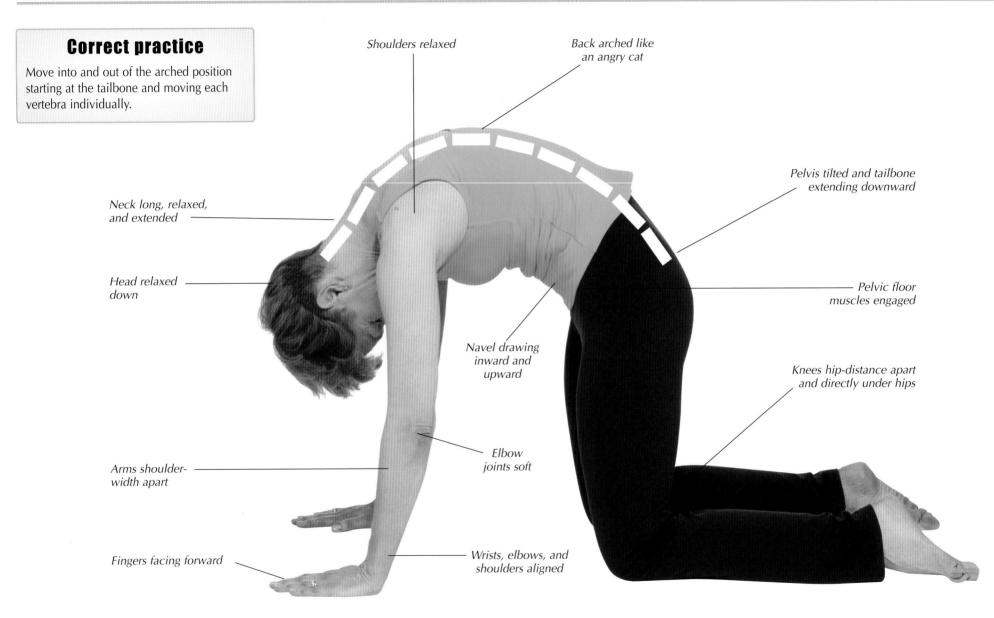

Shoulders relaxed

Back arched like an angry cat

Pelvis tilted and tailbone extending downward

Neck long, relaxed, and extended

Pelvic floor muscles engaged

Head relaxed down

Navel drawing inward and upward

Knees hip-distance apart and directly under hips

Elbow joints soft

Arms shoulder-width apart

Fingers facing forward

Wrists, elbows, and shoulders aligned

CAT STRETCH WITH ARM EXTENSION

By adding coordinated arm movement to the Cat Stretch you will improve your balance as well as your spine flexibility.

This is also a good exercise for strengthening the core muscles of the torso and adds a gentle stretch for the muscles in the shoulder area.

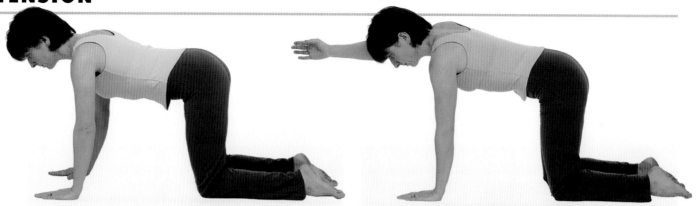

1 Kneel on all fours in neutral and check your alignment. **Inhale** slowly in this neutral position.

2 **As you exhale,** slowly raise your right arm out in front of you to shoulder height, keeping your right shoulder relaxed. Extend through the arm and out through the fingertips.

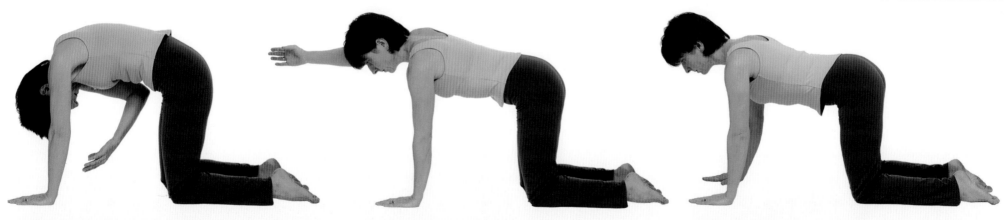

3 **As you inhale,** slowly arch your back into the cat position and bend the right elbow in to the waist. Remember to arch your back sequentially from the tailbone through the lower back, the middle back, then between the shoulder blades, and finally through the neck so that the head lengthens toward the floor as the spine arches.

4 **As you exhale,** extend your right arm back to shoulder height and uncurl. To uncurl, extend your tailbone back, followed by the lower back, the middle back, then between the shoulder blades, and through the neck. Extend the top of the head forward until you are back in neutral spine.

Repeat 3 times, following steps 3 and 4.

5 **As you inhale,** lower your arm and place your hand on the floor so you are back in the starting position.

Repeat 4 times with the left arm.

ALL FOURS LEG EXTENSIONS

This exercise focuses on maintaining neutral pelvis and spine while the leg is extending. It teaches economy of movement and core stability while strengthening the abdominal and back muscles.

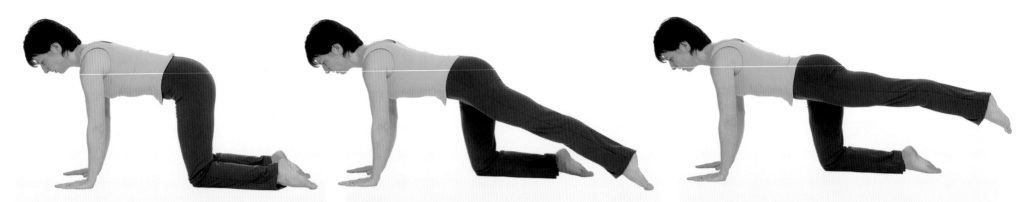

1 Kneel on all fours in neutral. Check that your joints are in alignment.

2 **As you inhale,** gently and smoothly extend your left leg along the floor in preparation.

3 **As you exhale,** lift your left leg to hip height. Draw the abdominal muscles up toward the spine as you lift.

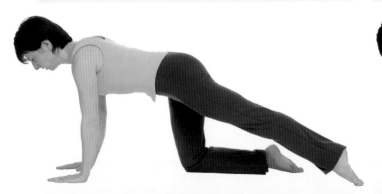

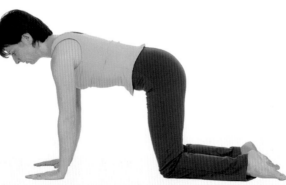

4 **As you inhale,** lower your left leg back down.

5 **As you exhale,** move your left leg back to neutral.

Repeat 6 times, following steps 2–5 and alternating legs.

Correct practice

When you are doing this exercise make sure that your torso stays still. Keep a quietness in the body by using the abdominal muscles to stabilize the lower back and pelvis as your leg is moving from the hip.

This stretch focuses on the oblique muscles responsible for rotating the body and bending sideways from the waist. These muscles, when strong, help to maintain good posture and streamline the body, giving you a sleeker waistline.

As the arm extends toward the ceiling, you will also feel a gentle stretch through the pectoral muscles of your chest. These muscles often get tight from hunching forward when sitting down.

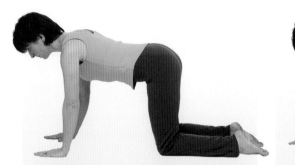 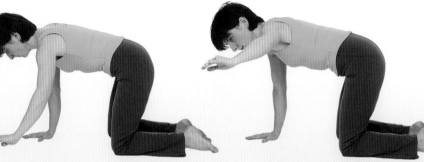 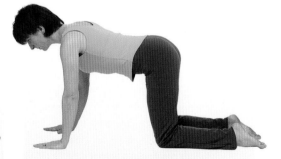

1 Kneel on all fours in neutral with joints aligned.

2 As you inhale, float your left arm out to the side and up toward the ceiling. Keep your shoulder and torso stable as you move your arm. Keep your pelvis in neutral.

3 As you exhale, rotate your chest and head by looking up into your left palm as it extends upward.

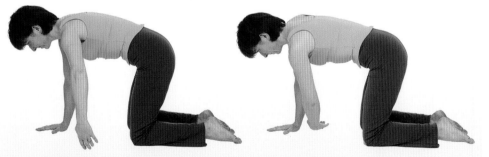 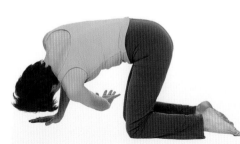

4 As you inhale, gently float your left arm back down toward the floor. Remember to keep your movements flowing smoothly with your breathing throughout the exercise.

5 As you exhale, reach your left arm between the right arm and leg. Let your head and neck relax.

Repeat 4–6 times, following steps 2–5.

6 As you inhale, float your arm back to the all fours position. **Exhale** in the neutral position.

Repeat 4–6 times with the right arm.

LATERAL STRETCH IN FOCUS

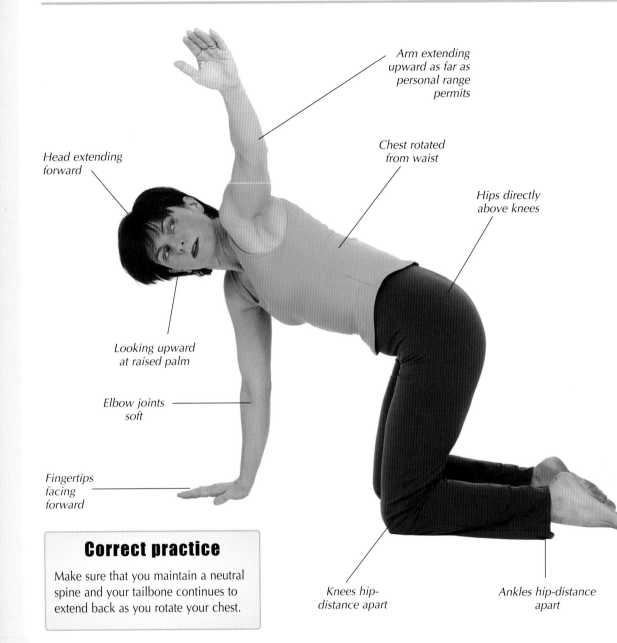

Arm extending upward as far as personal range permits

Chest rotated from waist

Head extending forward

Hips directly above knees

Looking upward at raised palm

Elbow joints soft

Fingertips facing forward

Knees hip-distance apart

Ankles hip-distance apart

Your personal range

Not everyone has the same range of movement; and it can differ on each side of your body.

To discover your range, rotate from the waist, keeping your focus on your hand. Keep your pelvis in neutral by making sure that both your hipbones are level and not rotating and that your tailbone is extending back. When you have rotated as far as you can, hold the position for a couple of breaths. Then see if you can extend the rotation a fraction more. Do not force the movement; allow your breathing to relax the muscles into the stretch.

Resting position

This stretch, called Child Pose, relaxes and stretches the spine. You can relax into this comfortable position after any exercise that works the spine. From a kneeling position, bring your buttocks down onto your heels, rest your forehead on the floor, and rest your arms by your sides. Inhale and exhale deeply to help gently stretch and relax your spine.

Correct practice

Make sure that you maintain a neutral spine and your tailbone continues to extend back as you rotate your chest.

Pilates exercises done in the all fours position are generally good for balance, and for giving your back more strength and flexibility. Only try this 8–10-minute flowing routine after you have mastered the individual exercises in this chapter, so you can confidently move from one exercise to the next.

Do some deep breathing on all fours before you begin, so you feel relaxed and well balanced in your neutral spine position. Then move through the routine slowly and gently, in time with your deep, rhythmic breathing.

Cat Stretch (page 75)

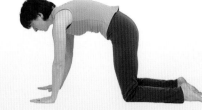 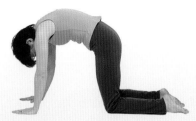

1 **Inhale** to prepare.

2 **Exhale**—arch spine, starting at tailbone and dropping head down last.

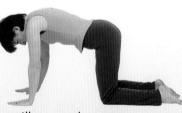 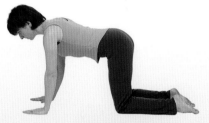

3 **Inhale**—uncurl back to neutral, starting with the tailbone and bringing head back up last.

Repeat 4 times.

Cat Stretch with Arm Extension (page 77)

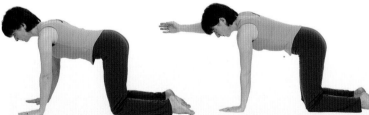
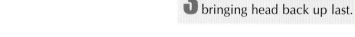
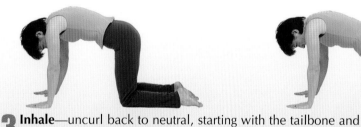
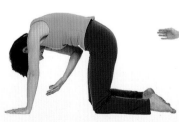 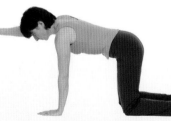 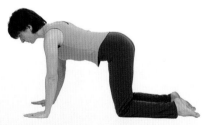

1 **Inhale** to prepare.

2 **Exhale**—raise right arm out in front to shoulder height.

3 **Inhale**—bend elbow in to waist and arch spine.

4 **Exhale**—uncurl back to neutral and extend arm.

Repeat 3 times, following steps 3 and 4.

5 **Inhale**—lower arm to starting position.

Repeat 4 times with left arm.

continued on next page

All Fours Leg Extensions (page 78)

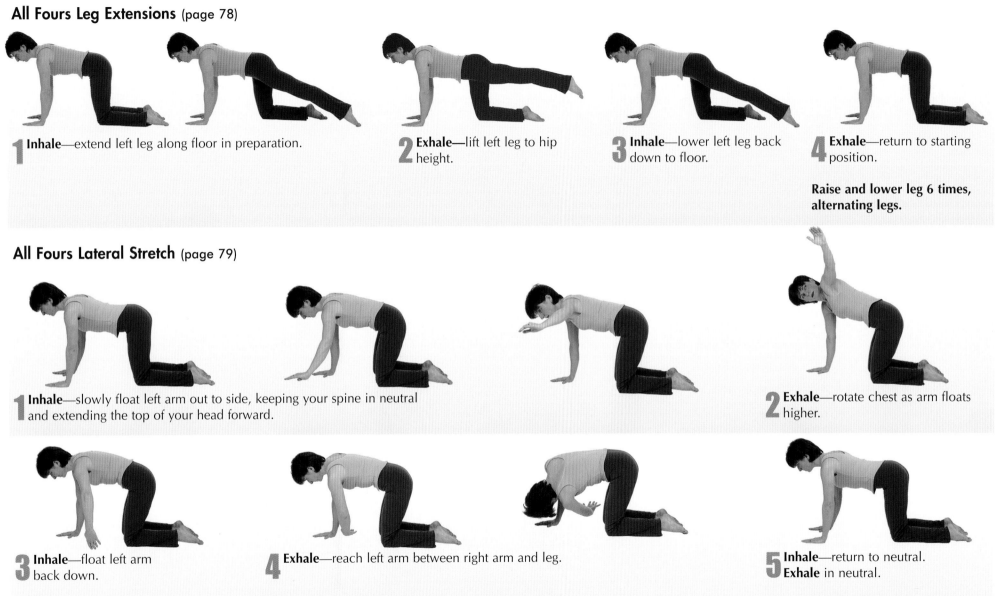

1 Inhale—extend left leg along floor in preparation.

2 Exhale—lift left leg to hip height.

3 Inhale—lower left leg back down to floor.

4 Exhale—return to starting position.

Raise and lower leg 6 times, alternating legs.

All Fours Lateral Stretch (page 79)

1 Inhale—slowly float left arm out to side, keeping your spine in neutral and extending the top of your head forward.

2 Exhale—rotate chest as arm floats higher.

3 Inhale—float left arm back down.

4 Exhale—reach left arm between right arm and leg.

Raise and lower left arm 4 times, repeating steps 1–4.

5 Inhale—return to neutral. Exhale in neutral.

Repeat 4 times with right arm.

Strong and Seated

About seated exercises

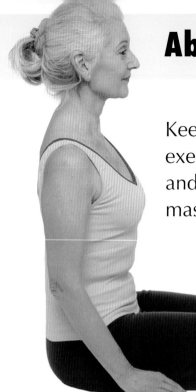

Keeping your spine in neutral while doing seated exercises is challenging. These exercises are demanding and an exciting extension to the movements you have mastered from previous chapters.

Most of us spend long periods each day sitting at a desk or in a car or train. Lengthy sitting encourages bad posture—the invention of the chair was truly detrimental to back health.

As children we were far more flexible because we spent time crawling, playing, and sitting on the floor. But as adults we spend more and more time sitting in chairs, which causes our hamstrings and back muscles to weaken and shorten.

Seated Pilates exercises are practiced sitting in good postural alignment with legs outstretched. This may feel uncomfortable at first, but as you develop strong and lengthened muscles sitting in neutral becomes easier.

Before trying out the seated exercises, review the neutral sitting position (see top right) and practice deep breathing. If you find any of the featured exercises too challenging at first, concentrate on lengthening your hamstrings.

Sitting in neutral

- Sit with your legs outstretched in front of you.

- Make sure your sitz bones are imprinting into the floor. If you are unsure, place your right hand under your right buttock and pull the flesh outward and to one side, then repeat on the other side. You should now be able to feel your sitz bones on the floor.

- Align your hips over your sitz bones and make sure your lower back keeps its natural curve.

- Lengthen up through your spine, aligning your shoulders directly over your hips.

- Float your chest upward without leaning back and check that your head is aligned over your shoulders.

Breathing practice

- **As you inhale** slowly and deeply, expand your ribcage sideways and backward, gently stretching the intercostal muscles.

- **As you exhale,** draw your navel in toward your spine, closing the front of your ribcage and drawing up through your pelvic floor muscles.

- Keep your pelvis in neutral and your shoulders relaxed while breathing.

CORRECT ALIGNMENT FOR SITTING

Postural problems often start from bad sitting habits. The exercises in this chapter will help you to improve your seated posture, an improvement that you should try to continue throughout the day.

Stretching your hamstrings will help you to position yourself in neutral for seated Pilates exercises. The exercise below is a good first step.

Gaze focused forward

Chin pulled back

Neck extending upward

Shoulders drawn down and aligned with hips

Chest floated upward

Spine upright and in neutral with natural spinal curves

Feet hip-distance apart

Knees, hips, and ankles in alignment

Hips directly over sitz bones and sitz bones imprinting into floor

Legs extending along floor

Hamstring stretch

1 Stand in neutral. Roll down as for the Full Roll-Down on page 39, **inhaling** and **exhaling** as you roll down. **Inhale** in the rolled-down position.

2 **As you exhale,** gently walk your hands two paces forward on the floor. Keep your legs straight, if you can, and place your palms flat on the floor.

3 Hold this position for 15 seconds, breathing slowly, and **ending on an exhale**. **Inhaling** and **exhaling,** slowly roll back up as for the Full Roll-Down.

The right way to sit

- **In a straight-back chair**—sit well back into the seat of an upright chair so that you can feel your buttocks resting against the chair back. Use the chair back to support your back. Make sure that your feet can touch the floor. Try not to slouch because this weakens your back muscles and restricts your circulation.

- **On a sofa**—never slouch into soft, unsupportive seating. This can disengage the muscles of the torso. Over time, this can cause backache. Sit as far back in the seat as possible and place a pillow under your buttocks or behind your back to give you more upright support.

- **In the car**—always adjust the seat to your back comfort; never sit in someone else's car seat position. An uncomfortable car seat can adversely affect your posture and cause back pain.

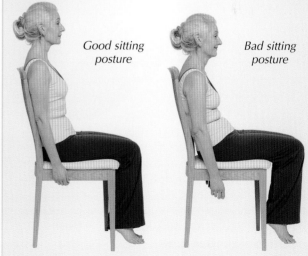

Good sitting posture

Bad sitting posture

85

MOBILIZING THE SPINE

This exercise focuses on lower back mobility. Try to feel the full length of your spine stretching as you round your back. Using your arms and hands in the exercise helps to lengthen the back muscles and move the spine into good alignment.

Correct practice

- Use your arms to increase your range of movement and support you as you inhale into the upright position.

- Tilt your pelvis when rounding the back to improve the range of movement in the lower back.

- Engage your pelvic floor muscles and draw the navel toward the spine as you exhale.

- Keep your shoulders relaxed—don't let them creep up to your ears as you exhale and round the back.

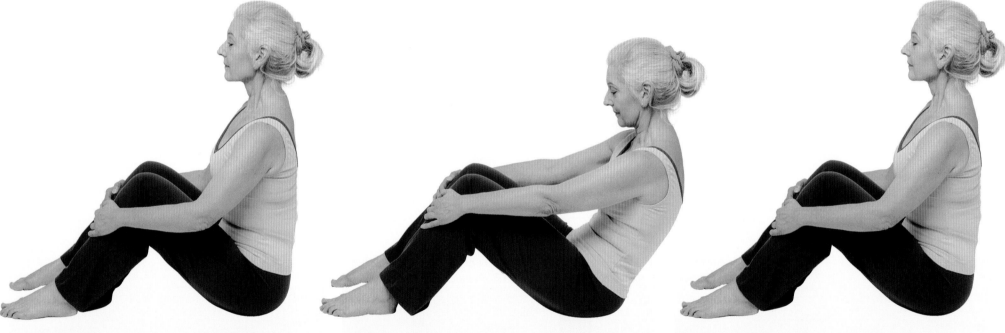

1 Sit right up on your sitz bones in neutral with your hips and shoulders in alignment. Bend your knees, making sure that your ankles, knees, and hips are in alignment. Place your hands around your shins just below the kneecap. Keep your elbows and shoulders relaxed and down. **As you inhale,** slowly lengthen upward through your torso.

2 **As you exhale,** slowly draw your navel toward your spine, engage your pelvic floor muscles, and hollow out through the center of your spine. Tilt your pelvis and round your back to lengthen the back muscles. Keep holding your legs as you round your back and lengthen through your arms.

3 **As you inhale,** slowly and gently release your pelvis and lengthen your torso back into the neutral spine position, remembering to draw your shoulders down.

Repeat 4–6 times in a slow, continuous, flowing movement.

Both of these exercises help to lengthen the hamstrings and calf muscles. They also focus on engaging the muscles of the back to maintain good spinal alignment. You may find them challenging and uncomfortable at first. If this is the case, use a cushion to sit on and start with just two or three repetitions until your muscles begin to lengthen and strengthen.

Rather than slouching in a chair watching TV, do the Flex and Point exercise. If you need extra support, rest the full length of your back against a wall.

Rounding Away—also called Seated Pelvic Tilt and Contraction—is performed with the legs lengthened along the floor and without the assistance of the arms. Use your Pilates ribcage breathing technique to assist you to control the movement. Move in time with your slow, deep breaths.

Flex and Point

1 Sit on the floor in neutral with your legs outstretched in front of you and the palms of your hands resting on the floor. **As you inhale,** slowly point your feet away from your torso.

2 As you exhale, draw your abdominal muscles in, engaging your pelvic floor muscles without clenching your buttocks, and flex your feet toward the ceiling. Keep your back in an upright, well-aligned position.

Repeat 4–6 times in a smooth, continuous movement.

Rounding Away

1 Sit on the floor in neutral with your legs outstretched in front of you and sitting up on your sitz bones. **As you inhale,** slowly point your feet away from your torso.

2 As you exhale, draw your navel toward your spine and engage your pelvic floor muscles. Tilt your pelvis and round your back to lengthen your back muscles (hollow out). At the same time, float your arms up to chest level and slightly lower your head.

As you exhale, return to neutral.

Repeat this step 4–6 times in a smooth, continuous movement.

This is another exercise that will lengthen your hamstrings and improve back mobility.

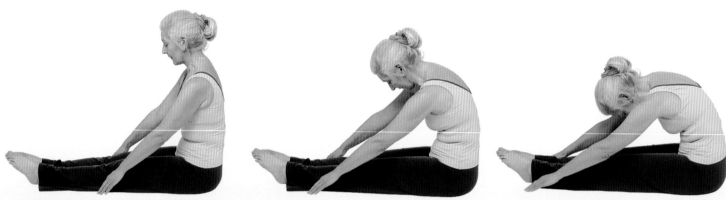

1 Sit on the floor in neutral with your legs outstretched in front of you and your hands on the floor beside you. Sit up on your sitz bones. **As you inhale,** lengthen your torso.

2 **As you exhale,** draw your navel in toward your spine, engaging your pelvic floor muscles and hollowing out through the center of your spine. At the same time, slowly slide your hands along the floor beside your thighs, extending yourself from your hip flexors. Imagine you have a beach ball

on your lap and you are rounding your back over it, forming your spine into a C-shape. Go as far forward as you can, keeping your legs fully extended along the floor. Try to keep your shoulders down and relaxed.

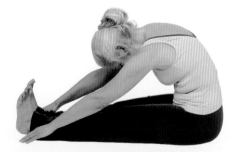

3 **As you inhale** in the forward extension, slowly flex your feet toward the ceiling and broaden the back of your ribcage.

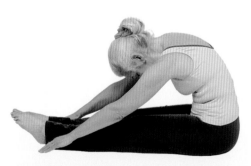

4 **As you exhale,** point your feet, drawing your navel in toward your spine, engaging the pelvic floor muscles, and hollowing out through the center.

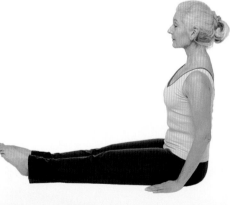

5 **As you inhale,** slowly uncurl your back to return to neutral.

Repeat 4–6 times.

Make it easier

If you have tight hamstrings, put a cushion under your buttocks to raise you off the floor a little. This will relieve the pull on the hamstrings.

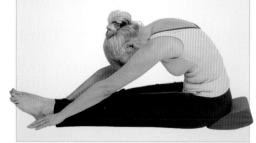

SPINAL ROTATION

This is the most challenging of the seated exercises in this chapter. To do it properly, you need a strong back, good control of your back and shoulder muscles, and lengthened hamstrings. You also need to be able to keep your pelvis well positioned.

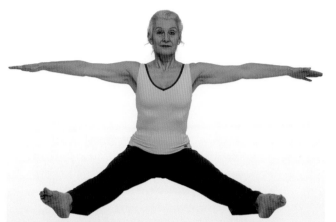

1 Sit in neutral with your legs outstretched and shoulder-width or slightly wider apart. Sit up on your sitz bones and raise your arms to shoulder height. **As you inhale,** slowly lengthen your torso upward.

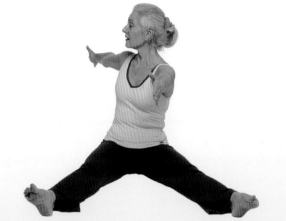

2 **As you exhale,** slowly rotate your ribcage from the waist to the right as far as you can without letting your shoulders or arms change their position. Let your shoulder girdle carry your arms.

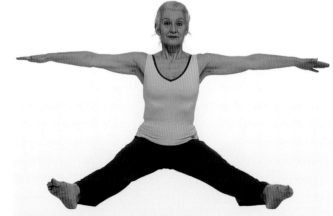

3 **As you inhale,** slowly and gently rotate back to the central position.

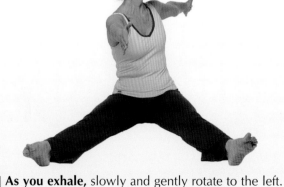

4 **As you exhale,** slowly and gently rotate to the left. Keep lengthening through the spine.

Make it easier

If your hamstrings are tight and weak, you may find it difficult to maintain this seated position while keeping your spine in neutral. Sitting on a cushion can make this easier.

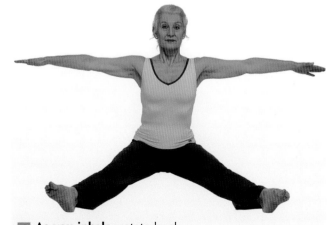

5 **As you inhale,** rotate back to the central position.

Repeat 4–6 times.

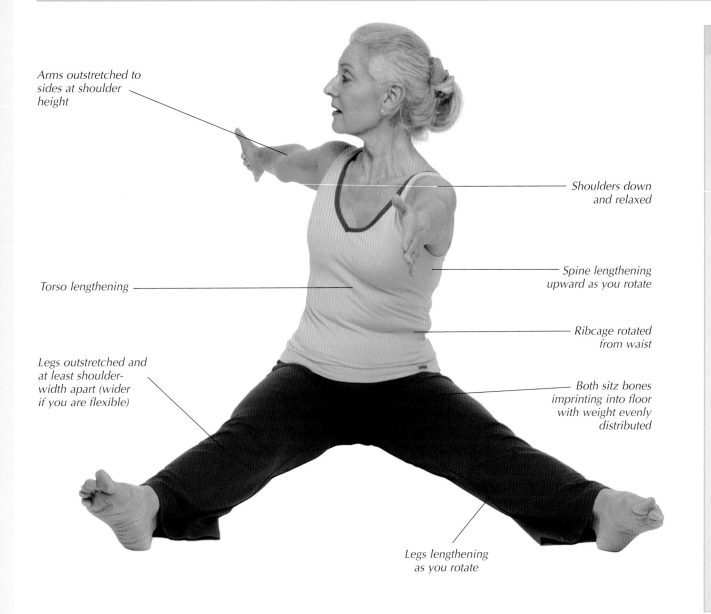

Arms outstretched to sides at shoulder height

Shoulders down and relaxed

Spine lengthening upward as you rotate

Torso lengthening

Ribcage rotated from waist

Legs outstretched and at least shoulder-width apart (wider if you are flexible)

Both sitz bones imprinting into floor with weight evenly distributed

Legs lengthening as you rotate

Common mistakes

Put a cushion under your buttocks and slightly bend your knees if your chest is collapsing and your lower back rounding like this.

The arms should be carried by the shoulder girdle as you rotate. Do not let your arms twist beyond the range of your shoulder joints or they may drop like this.

Beginners should practice the exercise routines in Chapters 4, 5, 6, and 7 several times to improve their Pilates technique before attempting this 8–10-minute seated routine.

When you are ready to start the routine, practice your deep ribcage breathing for a couple of minutes while seated in the first position for Mobilizing the Spine. As with all Pilates routines, once you begin, keep your movements slowly flowing in time with your breathing.

Mobilizing the Spine (page 86)

1 Sit with knees bent and hands around shins. **Inhale**—lengthen up through torso.

2 **Exhale**—tilt pelvis and round back.

3 **Inhale**—release pelvis and straighten spine to neutral.

Repeat 5 times.

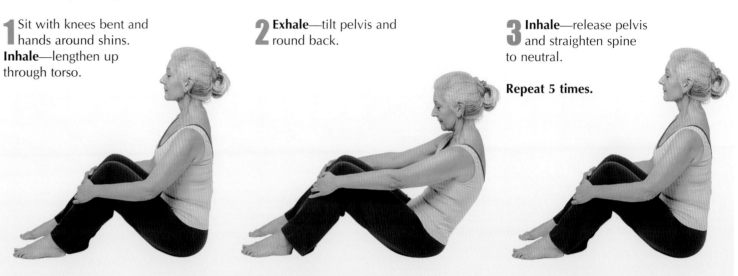

Flex and Point (page 87)

1 **Inhale**—point feet.

2 **Exhale**—flex feet toward ceiling.

Repeat 5 times.

Rounding Away (page 87)

1 **Inhale**—point feet.

2 **Exhale**—tilt pelvis, round back, and float arms to chest height, lowering head slightly.

Inhale—return to neutral.

Repeat 5 times.

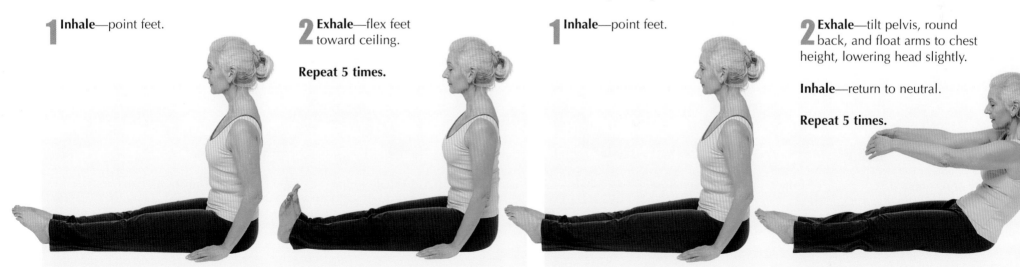

continued on next page

Sliding Hands to Toes (page 88)

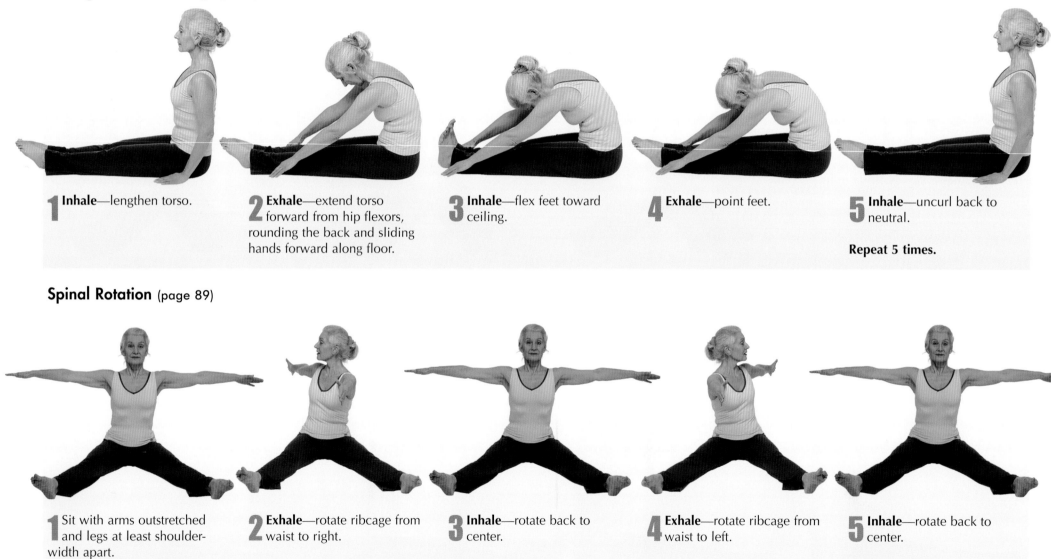

1 Inhale—lengthen torso.

2 Exhale—extend torso forward from hip flexors, rounding the back and sliding hands forward along floor.

3 Inhale—flex feet toward ceiling.

4 Exhale—point feet.

5 Inhale—uncurl back to neutral.

Repeat 5 times.

Spinal Rotation (page 89)

1 Sit with arms outstretched and legs at least shoulder-width apart.
Inhale—lengthen torso.

2 Exhale—rotate ribcage from waist to right.

3 Inhale—rotate back to center.

4 Exhale—rotate ribcage from waist to left.

5 Inhale—rotate back to center.

Repeat 5 times.

Deep Abdominal Exercises

About deep abdominal exercises

These exercises provide a strong challenge for the abdominal muscles. Make sure you are confident in your breathing technique and your control of the neutral spine position before starting them.

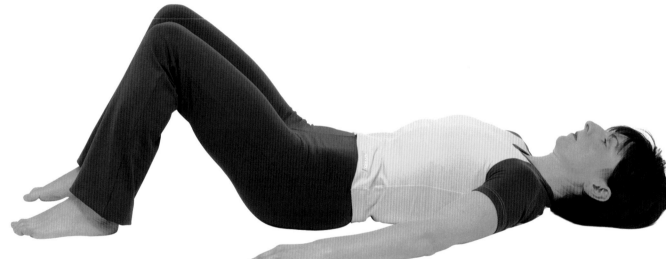

While exercises performed lying on your back may look easy, this can be deceptive, because the movements require both muscular strength and control. Try not to be over-ambitious at first. Follow the instructions carefully and use the tips and modifications. At the start, do fewer repetitions and focus on joint alignment and breathing.

These exercises will improve your core muscular strength and will help to streamline your body, giving you a longer, leaner look.

Don't forget to practice your breathing technique and check your neutral spine before you begin. Lying on your back is the most restful position for your spine and the easiest way to find neutral spine.

Lying on your back in neutral

- Lie on your back. Bend your knees and position your legs hip-distance apart so ankles, knees, and hips are in alignment. Place your feet flat on the floor facing forward in a parallel position, with your toes spread apart.

- Position your pelvis in neutral so that your lower back retains its natural curvature. Make sure your pubic bone and hipbones are level and your tailbone is extending toward your heels. Your sacrum should be imprinting into the floor.

- Imprint your upper spine and shoulder blades into the floor and relax your arms.

- Keep your shoulders relaxed and drawing away from your neck.

- Lengthen through the muscles of the neck and extend the top of your head along the floor.

Breathing practice

- **As you inhale,** feel your shoulders relax and the back of your ribcage imprint deeper into the floor as your ribcage expands sideways and backward.

- **As you exhale,** feel the front of your ribcage drawing in and down. The apex of the ribs should be closing together. At the same time, draw your abdominal muscles inward and upward toward the ribs.

The neck and shoulder area is where many people hold stress, especially when they are tired, worried, or have jobs that involve sitting for long periods. When your neck and shoulder muscles are stressed, your shoulders start to hunch. This will gradually lead to weak, tight muscles, headaches, and back pain.

Releasing tension from the neck and shoulders with simple mobility exercises like this helps improve your posture and relieve everyday aches and pains.

Neck alignment

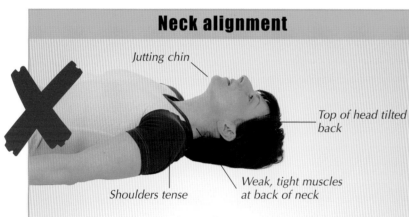

Jutting chin

Top of head tilted back

Weak, tight muscles at back of neck

Shoulders tense

You may need to put a thin pillow under your head to find the correct neutral position. A pillow will help to correct the alignment of the neck so that you can retrain the muscles to lengthen.

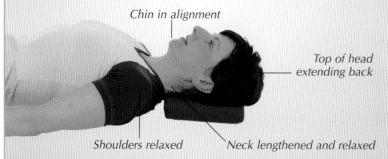

Chin in alignment

Top of head extending back

Shoulders relaxed

Neck lengthened and relaxed

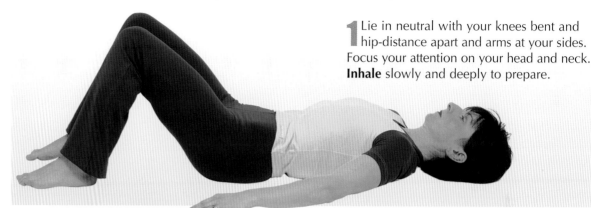

1 Lie in neutral with your knees bent and hip-distance apart and arms at your sides. Focus your attention on your head and neck. **Inhale** slowly and deeply to prepare.

2 **As you exhale,** slowly draw your chin down toward your chest, lengthening the muscles at the back of your neck without lifting your head from the floor.

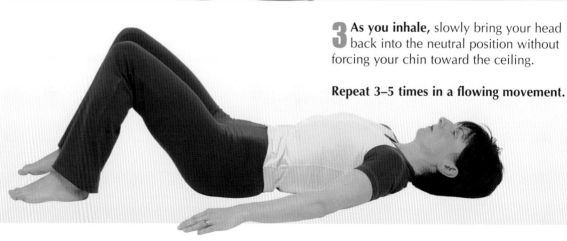

3 **As you inhale,** slowly bring your head back into the neutral position without forcing your chin toward the ceiling.

Repeat 3–5 times in a flowing movement.

For good posture you need abdominal strength to support your back, maintain spinal alignment, and hold your joints in the correct position. In traditional fitness classes "sit-ups" are often done to strengthen the rectus abdominus muscle, more commonly known as the "six pack." This muscle enables you to curl your head and legs toward your stomach when lying on your back, but it is not attached to the spine, so does not help to improve your posture. Because it is a fashionable muscle rather than a functional one, it is often over-exercised to give the outward curves of rippling muscle so popular with men. However, if the rectus abdominus is exercised incorrectly, it can lead to a firm but pot belly and unbalanced posture.

Pilates exercises focus on the transversus muscle, which is attached to the upper spine and runs horizontally around the center of the abdomen. Because it is connected to the spine, this muscle is much more important for core stability than the rectus abdominus.

Chest Floating in the supine position works the transversus and the rectus abdominus muscles together, promoting a more balanced and properly aligned spine.

1 Lie on your back in neutral with your knees bent and your ankles, knees, and hips in alignment. Check your pelvic alignment and relax your shoulders. With your elbows bent, place your hands at the back of your head to support its weight. **Inhale** slowly to prepare.

2 **As you exhale,** slowly float your chest, neck, and head toward the ceiling, keeping the weight of your head in your hands. Your neck and shoulders should remain in alignment with your head as your chest floats upward. When you have floated up as far as you can, hold the position and **inhale** slowly.

3 **As you exhale,** gently and smoothly lower your chest, neck, and head back down to neutral.

Repeat 4–6 times in a smooth, continuous movement.

On the exhale...

- Make sure your abdominal muscles draw inward and upward toward your ribs, making a hollow through your center without tilting the pelvis as you lift your chest.

- Draw your ribs inward and down as you exhale so your ribs aren't pushing up to the ceiling but are stabilizing the upper back and engaging the transversus muscle.

- Use your abdominal muscles as a drawbridge to lift the chest, neck, and shoulders.

- Don't lift so high or repeat so many times if you find it difficult to retain the hollow through the abdominal muscles.

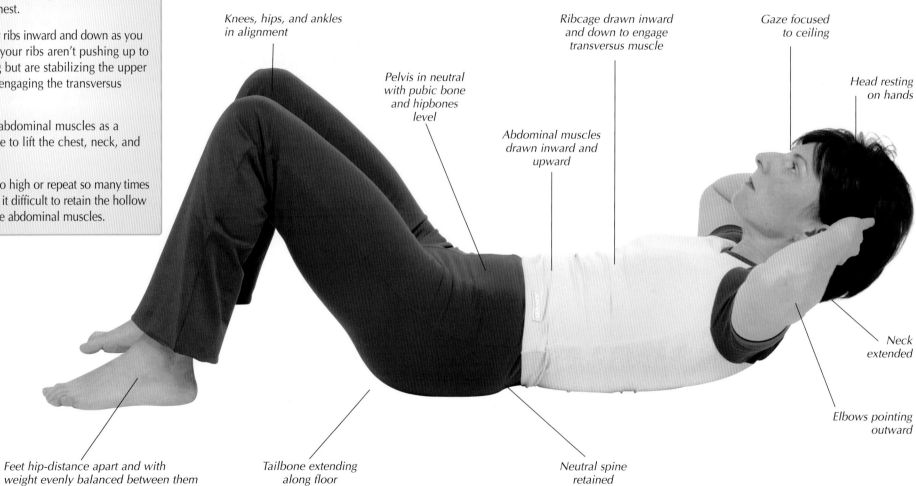

Knees, hips, and ankles in alignment

Ribcage drawn inward and down to engage transversus muscle

Gaze focused to ceiling

Pelvis in neutral with pubic bone and hipbones level

Head resting on hands

Abdominal muscles drawn inward and upward

Neck extended

Elbows pointing outward

Feet hip-distance apart and with weight evenly balanced between them

Tailbone extending along floor

Neutral spine retained

If you want the ultimate flat stomach, then this is the exercise that will give it to you! It may look like a crunch or sit-up that most people are familiar with, but the Cervical Curl is quite different. It focuses on the transversus muscle, which acts as a lever to lift the head, neck, and upper chest while keeping the pelvis in neutral. This muscle engagement, combined with the deep ribcage breathing, develops a flat, firm abdominal wall.

The Cervical Curl not only focuses on strengthening your abdominal muscles but also on strengthening your neck muscles. You often see people doing sit-ups by pulling on their necks and using their shoulders to lift themselves. This creates a lot of tension on the neck and does not give enough focus to the deep muscles of the torso.

Correct practice

• Make sure your pelvis stays in neutral and does not tilt, forcing the lumbar spine into the floor.

• Keep your ankles, knees, and hips in alignment by pressing gently down through your feet.

• Stop your shoulders from rounding by keeping your fingertips on the floor.

1 Lie on your back in neutral with your knees bent and arms at your sides. Check your neutral pelvis position and your ankle, knee, and hip alignment. **Inhale,** expanding the ribs sideways and backward.

2 **As you exhale,** lengthen your arms, slide your fingertips along the floor, and draw your shoulders away from your head. Contract your abdominal muscles inward and upward, closing the ribcage. Curl your head, neck, chest, and shoulders off the floor. Let your chin lower slightly, drawing your head back to keep your neck muscles lengthened. **Inhale** in the lifted position, keeping your shoulders stable. **As you exhale,** float your head, neck, and chest back down to the floor.

Repeat 4–6 times in a slow, flowing movement.

Tight hamstrings combined with weak hip flexors can restrict movement in the lower back and pelvic area. This exercise works on lengthening your hamstrings while you maintain a neutral pelvis position. It also improves abdominal and hip flexor strength.

If you find it challenging because your hamstrings are tight, follow the tips on the right.

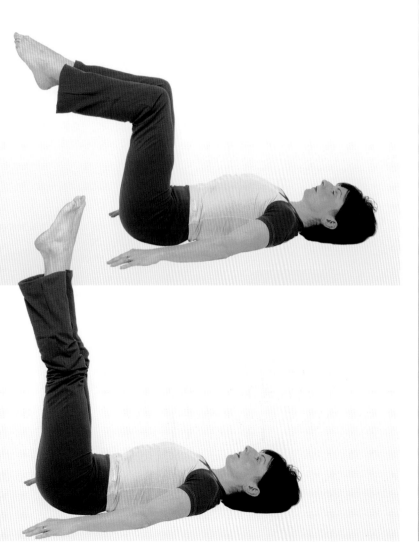

1 Lie in neutral with your head, neck, and shoulders resting on the floor and your arms at your sides. Float one knee at a time to a right-angle position so that your knees are bent and directly over your hips and your ankles form a horizontal line with your knees. **Inhale** slowly in this position, breathing into the back of your ribcage without tensing your shoulders.

2 **As you exhale,** extend both legs toward the ceiling, keeping your ankles and knees over your hip joints. Draw your abdominal muscles inward and upward as you extend your legs and keep the front of your ribcage stable.
As you inhale, bring your legs back to the right-angle position.

Repeat 4–6 times in a slow, continuous movement.

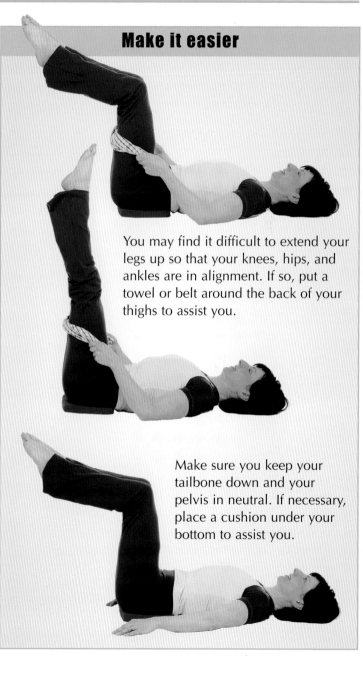

Make it easier

You may find it difficult to extend your legs up so that your knees, hips, and ankles are in alignment. If so, put a towel or belt around the back of your thighs to assist you.

Make sure you keep your tailbone down and your pelvis in neutral. If necessary, place a cushion under your bottom to assist you.

This challenging exercise works the shoulder blades, hip flexors, and core stability. Make sure you have mastered the Cervical Curl (page 98) before moving on to this exercise.

To help you coordinate the movement, plan ahead. Think "contraction" before the action on the exhale so that you engage your muscles and stabilize your torso before you reach the extreme position (step 2). The leg extension and the torso curl should work together as a team.

Make it easier

- Put a thin pillow under your pelvic area if your lower back aches or if you experience discomfort from your sacrum pressing into the floor.
- Try extending your leg toward the ceiling instead of parallel to the floor if your lower back arches when you extend.

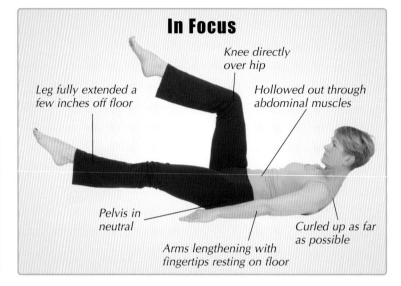

In Focus

Leg fully extended a few inches off floor

Knee directly over hip

Hollowed out through abdominal muscles

Pelvis in neutral

Arms lengthening with fingertips resting on floor

Curled up as far as possible

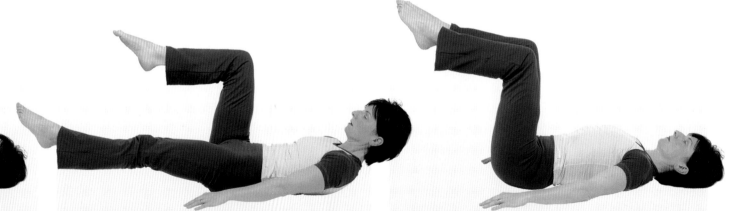

1 Lie on your back in neutral. Raise both legs so that ankles, knees, and hips form a right angle, with the knees directly above the hips. Keep head, neck, and shoulders on the floor with your hands by your sides. **Inhale** slowly in this neutral spine position to prepare.

2 **As you exhale,** slowly curl your head, neck, and shoulders off the floor. At the same time, slowly extend your left leg. Keep your fingertips on the floor and reach your arms along the floor, relaxing and drawing the shoulders down and away from the neck. **Inhale** slowly in the curled position.

3 **As you exhale,** slowly draw your leg back to the right-angle position and, at the same time, lower your head, neck, and chest back down.

Repeat 4–6 times, alternating the legs.

SINGLE LEG EXTENSIONS

This is an advanced version of Single Leg Extensions with Cervical Curl (see page 100). The movement is quicker than that in most Pilates exercises, so good technique is important. The exercise focuses on endurance and uses a different breathing pattern. If your neck and shoulders start to ache, exercise with your head and shoulders on the floor and your legs extending more toward the ceiling.

> **CAUTION: If you experience any sharp pain, dizziness, faintness, or tingling in your shoulders or arms, stop this exercise immediately.**

Make it easier

- Put a thin pillow under your pelvic area if your lower back aches or if you experience discomfort from your sacrum pressing into the floor.

- Try extending your leg toward the ceiling instead of out in front of you if you find that your lower back is arching.

- Place one hand at the back of your head if your neck aches.

- Do only as many extensions as you can while still holding good postural alignment.

1 Lie on your back in neutral with your head on the floor, legs lifted into the right-angle position, arms relaxed at your sides, and shoulders drawing away from your ears. **Inhale** slowly to prepare.

2 **As you exhale,** curl your head, neck, shoulders, and chest away from the floor, sliding your fingertips along the floor. When you have curled as far as you can, hold that position.
As you inhale, slowly extend your left leg, keeping the right leg at a right angle.

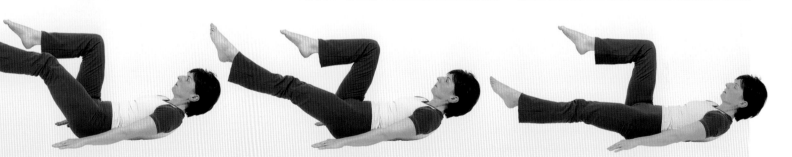

3 **As you exhale,** change legs. Keep changing legs with each "mini" exhale in a panting fashion. When you have expelled all the air, **inhale** then **exhale** continuing the movement. The movement should be fast and continuous.

Repeat, changing legs 5–10 times.

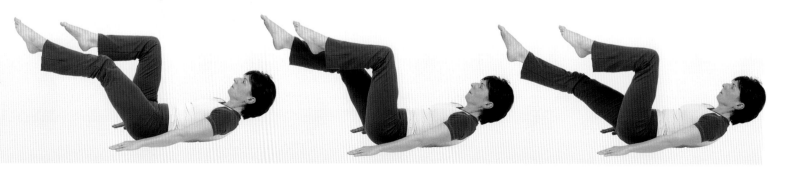

Like the Knee Sways on page 51, this rotation exercise releases tension from the middle of the back and stretches the waist and sides of the body. It also helps to strengthen the deep core muscles. This version of Knee Sways is more challenging because it requires a lot more stability work from the core muscles of the torso.

Correct practice

- Make sure your knees are directly over your hips and your feet are in alignment with your knees, forming a right angle.

- Keep both shoulders relaxed and on the floor. As you sway to the right, your left shoulder will try to lift and vice versa. Let your shoulders be your guide—only sway your legs as far as you can without your shoulders lifting.

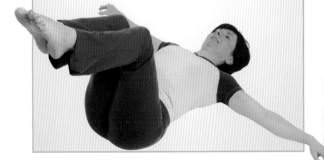

1 Lie on your back in neutral. Keeping your knees and ankles together as if they were one leg, lift them to a right-angle position. Spread your arms out on the floor at about shoulder height. Make sure your head, neck, and shoulders are relaxed on the floor—put a pillow under your head if you need one. **Inhale** slowly and deeply into the upper back to prepare.

2 As you exhale, pull your abdominal muscles in and sway your knees and right hip over to the left side as far as you can without letting the right shoulder lift off the floor. Keep your knees and ankles together.
Inhale slowly in this position.

3 As you exhale, slowly bring your knees back up to their raised, right-angle position. Keep your gaze focused upward to the ceiling.
Inhale slowly in this neutral position.

4 As you exhale, sway your knees to the right, checking that the left shoulder is imprinting into the floor.
Inhale slowly in this position.
As you exhale, bring your knees back to the center. Keep your gaze focused upward to the ceiling.

Repeat 4–6 times in a flowing movement.

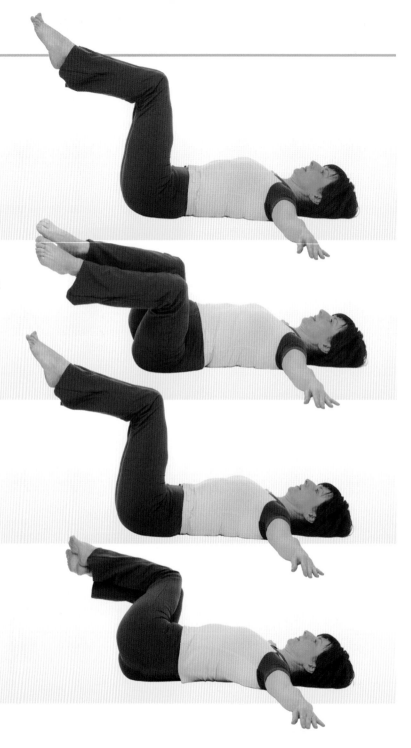

Here's a good Pilates routine if you are aiming for a longer, leaner look. It combines all the exercises you will have learned in this chapter. Refer back to the detailed instructions if you need a refresher course in any of the exercises.

Keep your movements flowing from one exercise to the next for a 10–12-minute routine. Remember to move slowly and evenly in time with your deep breathing.

Cervical Nod—Supine (page 95)

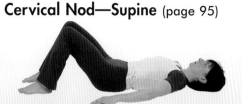 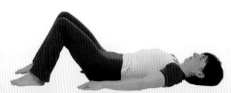 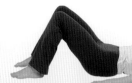

1 Inhale to prepare.

2 Exhale—draw chin down toward chest.

3 Inhale—bring head back to neutral.

Repeat 3 times.

Chest Floating—Supine (page 96)

 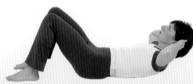 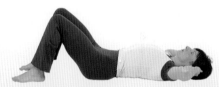

1 Inhale to prepare, with weight of head in hands.

2 Exhale—float chest, neck, and head toward ceiling. **Inhale.**

3 Exhale—lower chest, neck, and head.

Repeat 4–6 times.

Cervical Curl (page 98)

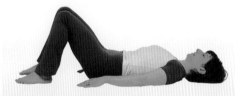 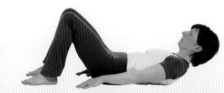 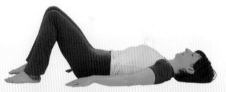

1 Inhale to prepare.

2 Exhale—slide fingers along floor and curl head, neck, chest, and shoulders. **Inhale.**

3 Exhale—lower head back down.

Repeat 4–6 times.

Leg Extensions from Right Angle (page 99)

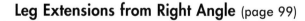 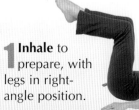 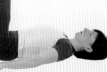

1 Inhale to prepare, with legs in right-angle position.

2 Exhale—extend both legs toward ceiling.

3 Inhale—bring legs back to right angle.

Repeat 4–6 times.

continued on next page

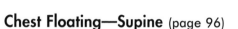 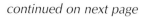

EXERCISE ROUTINE—WORKING THE DEEP ABDOMINALS (continued)

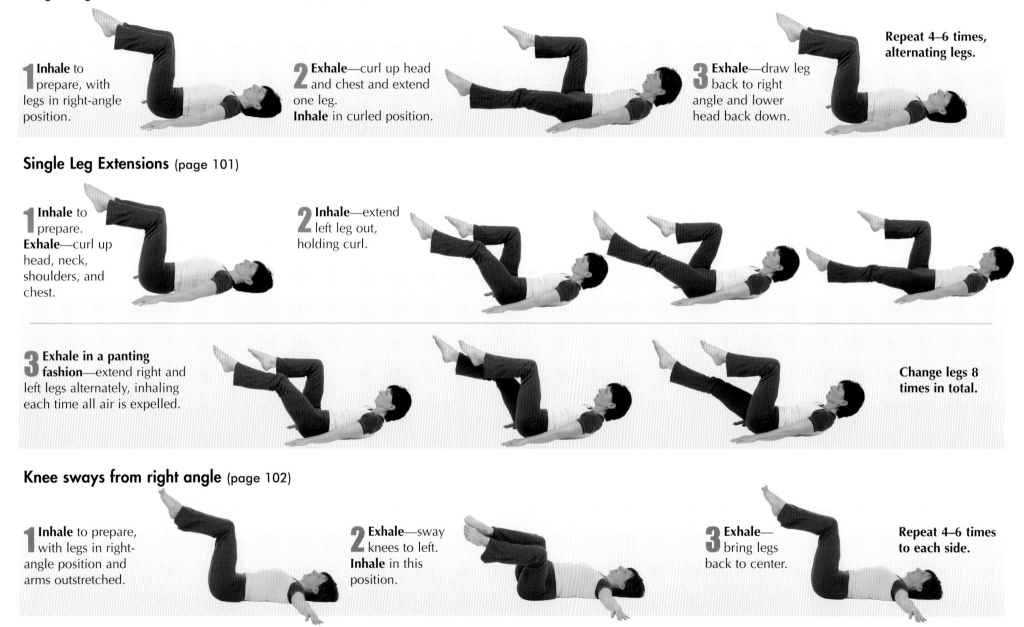

Single Leg Extensions with Cervical Curl (page 100)

1 **Inhale** to prepare, with legs in right-angle position.

2 **Exhale**—curl up head and chest and extend one leg.
Inhale in curled position.

3 **Exhale**—draw leg back to right angle and lower head back down.

Repeat 4–6 times, alternating legs.

Single Leg Extensions (page 101)

1 **Inhale** to prepare.
Exhale—curl up head, neck, shoulders, and chest.

2 **Inhale**—extend left leg out, holding curl.

3 **Exhale in a panting fashion**—extend right and left legs alternately, inhaling each time all air is expelled.

Change legs 8 times in total.

Knee sways from right angle (page 102)

1 **Inhale** to prepare, with legs in right-angle position and arms outstretched.

2 **Exhale**—sway knees to left.
Inhale in this position.

3 **Exhale**—bring legs back to center.

Repeat 4–6 times to each side.

Fast-Track Workout

About the fast-track workout

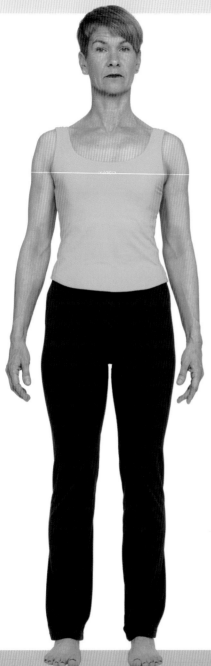

This workout brings the exercises you have learned in Chapters 2–9 into a flowing routine. It will help you to refine your Pilates techniques.

Every time you practice Pilates, you are gently re-educating your body, moving it away from its old habits and developing your own personal body awareness.

Having practiced many of the exercises in the book, this workout will add another dimension to the way you can challenge your body with Pilates. It links, in a flowing succession, exercises performed in different positions to take you to a new level.

This workout should take about 15 minutes and can easily fit into a busy schedule. It can be performed at any time during the day when you have a little time to spare.

The workout starts with a warm-up in the standing position. As with all Pilates exercises, check your posture before beginning. Make sure your ankles, knees, and hips are in alignment and that your weight is evenly distributed. Position your pelvis in neutral,

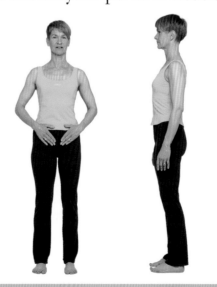

using your fingertips to check your alignment.

Once standing in neutral, align your neck with your shoulders. To do this, jut your chin forward and then draw it in so your neck is lengthening and you feel that you are lifting from the top of your head.

Breathing exercise

In a well-aligned standing position, practice your deep breathing before you start your warm-up.

The workout instructions in this section are given in abbreviated form. If you need more detailed reminders turn back to the main instructions for each exercise (the page number is given in the heading).

Remember to breathe through each movement in the exercises and to keep the exercises gently flowing.

Knee Bends (page 36)

1 Stand in neutral.

2 **Inhale**—bend your knees, keeping your heels on the floor. Allow hip flexors to relax so that your pelvis stays in neutral. Shoulders remain over your hips.

3 **Exhale**—straighten your legs, pressing heels into the floor, extending the tailbone down, contracting the pelvic floor muscles, and pulling the abdominal muscles in and up.

Repeat 6 times.

Pelvic Rock (page 37)

1 Stand in neutral with your knees slightly bent.

2 **Inhale**—tilt your pelvis as far forward as you can.

3 **Exhale**—tilt your pelvis as far back as you can.

Repeat 6–8 times.

Full Roll-Down (page 39)

1 Stand in neutral.

2 **Inhale**—curl your head forward and roll down through the neck, shoulders, and upper back, bending the knees as your shoulders pass your waist.

3 **Exhale**—roll down, keeping head, neck, shoulders, and arms relaxed and knees slightly bent.

4 **Inhale**—start uncurling through the lower back.

5 **Exhale**—uncurl through the upper back and neck, bringing the head up into alignment.

Repeat 4–6 times.

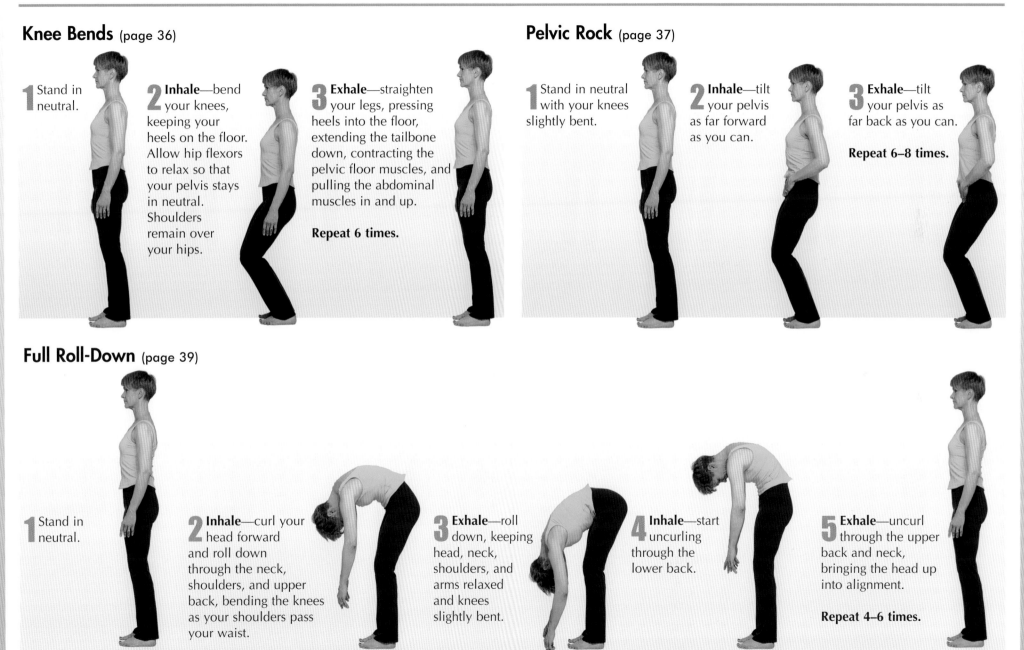

continued on next page

Lateral Stretch
(page 41)

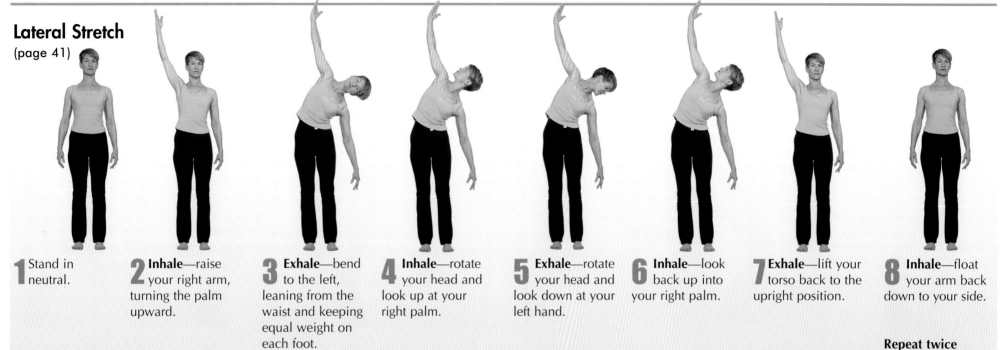

1 Stand in neutral.

2 Inhale—raise your right arm, turning the palm upward.

3 Exhale—bend to the left, leaning from the waist and keeping equal weight on each foot.

4 Inhale—rotate your head and look up at your right palm.

5 Exhale—rotate your head and look down at your left hand.

6 Inhale—look back up into your right palm.

7 Exhale—lift your torso back to the upright position.

8 Inhale—float your arm back down to your side.

Repeat twice on each side.

Cat Stretch (page 75)

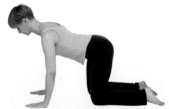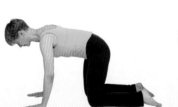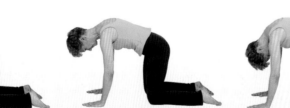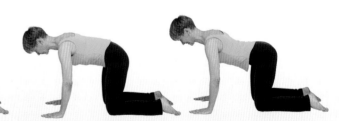

1 Kneel on all fours in neutral. **Inhale** to prepare.

2 Exhale—arch your spine, starting at the tailbone. Tilt the pelvis back, then round the lower back, the middle back, through the shoulder blades, neck, and head. **Inhale** in this arched position.

3 Exhale—extend tailbone, then roll down through the lower back, middle back, upper back, and neck. Extend the top of your head and engage the abdominal muscles to return to neutral.

Repeat 4 or 5 times.

continued on next page

Opposite Arm and Leg Extensions (page 129)

1 Kneel in neutral.

2 Inhale—extend your right arm and left leg along the floor.

3 Exhale—lift your arm and leg to shoulder and hip height, drawing the abdominal muscles up toward the spine.

4 Inhale—lower your arm and leg back down.

5 Exhale—bring arm and leg back to neutral.

Repeat 6 times on each side.

All Fours Lateral Stretch (page 79)

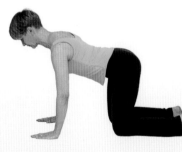

1 Kneel in neutral.

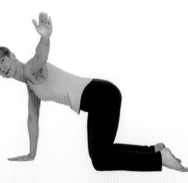

2 Inhale—float left arm out to the side.
Exhale—as your arm extends up toward the ceiling, rotate your chest and head to look up into your palm.

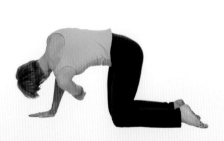

3 Inhale—float your arm down toward the floor.
Exhale—reach your left arm between the right arm and leg, let your head and neck relax, and rotate from the waist to keep in neutral.

Repeat 4–6 times on one side, then 4–6 times on other side.

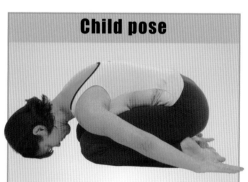

Child pose

Now, stretch your spine before continuing. Rest your buttocks on your heels, your forehead on the floor, and your arms by your sides with your hands palms up.

Inhale and exhale deeply 4–6 times, gently stretching the spine.

continued on next page

FAST-TRACK WORKOUT (continued)

Spinal Rotation
(page 89)

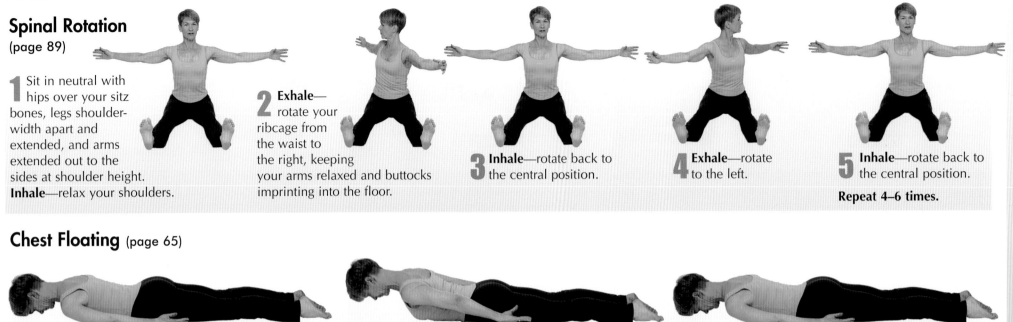

1 Sit in neutral with hips over your sitz bones, legs shoulder-width apart and extended, and arms extended out to the sides at shoulder height. **Inhale**—relax your shoulders.

2 **Exhale**—rotate your ribcage from the waist to the right, keeping your arms relaxed and buttocks imprinting into the floor.

3 **Inhale**—rotate back to the central position.

4 **Exhale**—rotate to the left.

5 **Inhale**—rotate back to the central position.

Repeat 4–6 times.

Chest Floating (page 65)

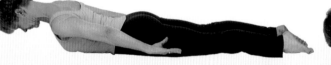 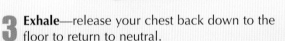

1 Move onto your front in neutral with the tip of your nose on the floor, arms extending, legs outstretched, and ankles, knees, and hips in alignment. **Inhale** to prepare.

2 **Exhale**—draw the abdominals in, hollow out the belly, and float the chest off the floor. Keep head, neck, and shoulders aligned. Extend your arms, keeping the shoulders relaxed and pelvis in neutral. **Inhale** in this position.

3 **Exhale**—release your chest back down to the floor to return to neutral.

Repeat 4–6 times.

Single Leg Lift (page 64)

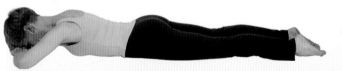 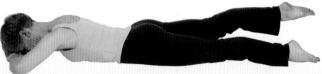 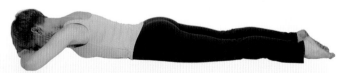

1 Lie on your front, with your hands under your forehead, shoulders relaxed, and ankles, knees, and hips in alignment. **Inhale** to prepare.

2 **Exhale**—draw the abdominals in, hollowing out the belly, and lengthen and lift one leg off the floor. Keep both hipbones on the floor.

3 **Inhale**—lower your leg back to the floor to return to neutral.

Repeat 4–6 times, alternating legs.

continued on next page

Quad and Hip Flexor Stretch (page 70)

Lie on your front in neutral with legs together. Bend the right knee and hold your ankle with your right hand or with a towel wrapped around it. Place your left hand under your forehead. Imprint your pubic bone and hipbones into the floor and lengthen the tailbone toward the heels. Relax your shoulders and chest.

Inhale—to prepare.
Exhale—draw the abdominals in. Tilt your pelvis to imprint the pubic and hipbones into the floor.
Inhale—hold the stretch.
Exhale—deepen the pelvic tilt to increase the stretch.
Inhale—release.

Repeat with left leg.

The Bridge (page 49)

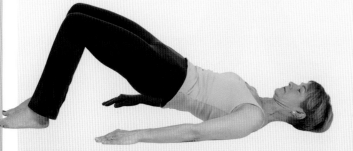

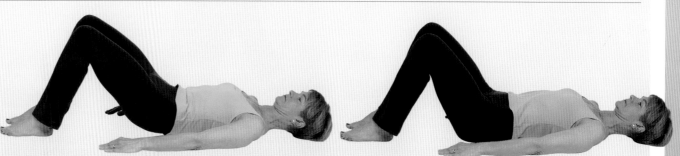

1 Turn over onto your back and lie in neutral with your knees bent and hip-distance apart. **Inhale** to prepare.

2 **Exhale**—tilt your pelvis so that your pubic bone tilts toward your navel, then peel your vertebrae off the floor, one at a time, until your body is resting on your

shoulder blades. Press down through your feet as you curl up, engaging the inner thighs. Keep shoulders relaxed and arms reaching along the floor.

3 **Inhale** in this raised position.

4 **Exhale**—lower the back, working down through the spine, imprinting the vertebrae, one at a time, until the tailbone touches down.

Repeat 4–6 times.

continued on next page

Single-Leg Knee Floating (page 52)

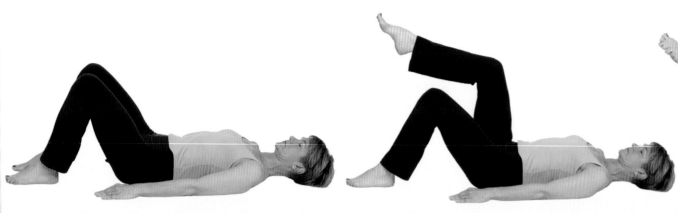

1 Lie on your back in neutral with your knees bent and hip-distance apart. **Inhale** to prepare.

2 **Exhale**—using only the hip flexors, float your right leg up to a right angle with the knee over the hip. **Inhale** in this position.

Resting pose

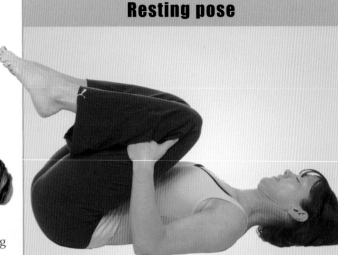

To stretch your spine between exercises when lying on your back, bring your knees to your chest and with your hands, gently pull the back of your thighs closer to your chest. **Inhale and exhale deeply 4–6 times** to relax and stretch the spine.

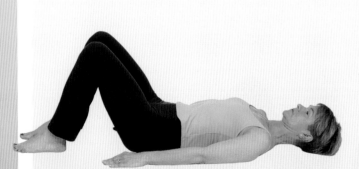

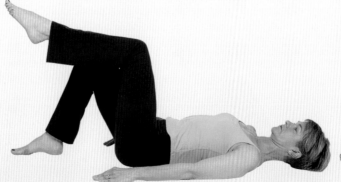

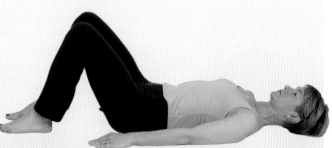

3 **Exhale**—float your foot back down, drawing down through the ribs and contracting your abdominals. **Inhale** to prepare.

4 **Exhale**—float your left leg up to a right angle. **Inhale** in this position.

5 **Exhale**—float your leg back down.

Repeat 6 times.

continued on next page

Leg Extensions from Right Angle
(page 99)

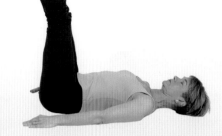
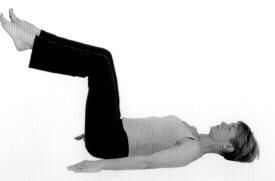

1 Lie on your back in neutral with arms at your sides. Float one knee at a time up to the right-angle position, with your knees over your hips. **Inhale** to prepare.

2 **Exhale**—extend both legs upward, keeping ankles and knees over hips and drawing abdominals in.

3 **Inhale**—lower your legs back to the right-angle position.

Repeat 4–6 times.

Cervical Curl (page 98)

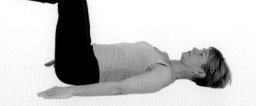

1 Lie on your back in neutral, with knees bent. **Inhale** to prepare.

2 **Exhale**—contract the abdominal muscles and curl the head, neck, chest, and shoulders off the floor, sliding fingertips along the floor and drawing shoulders away from the head. **Inhale** in the lifted position.

3 **Exhale**—float the chest back down to neutral.

Repeat 4–6 times.

Single Leg Extensions with Cervical Curl
(page 100)

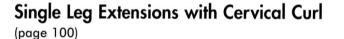
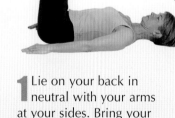

1 Lie on your back in neutral with your arms at your sides. Bring your legs up to the right-angle position with your knees over your hips. **Inhale** to prepare.

2 **Exhale**—slowly curl your head, neck, and shoulders off the floor and extend your left leg out in front of you. Keep your fingertips on the floor as your arms lengthen. **Inhale** in the lifted position.

3 **Exhale**—draw your leg back to the right-angle position and lower your chest back down.

Repeat 4–6 times, alternating legs.

continued on next page

Knee Sways from Right Angle (page 102)

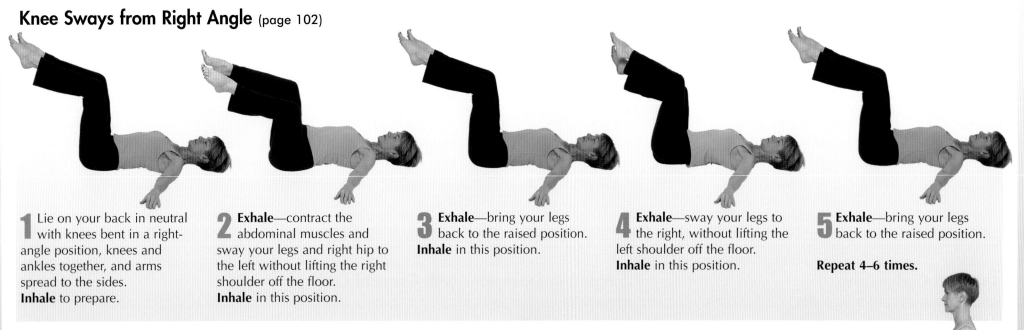

1 Lie on your back in neutral with knees bent in a right-angle position, knees and ankles together, and arms spread to the sides. **Inhale** to prepare.

2 **Exhale**—contract the abdominal muscles and sway your legs and right hip to the left without lifting the right shoulder off the floor. **Inhale** in this position.

3 **Exhale**—bring your legs back to the raised position. **Inhale** in this position.

4 **Exhale**—sway your legs to the right, without lifting the left shoulder off the floor. **Inhale** in this position.

5 **Exhale**—bring your legs back to the raised position.

Repeat 4–6 times.

Chest Floating—Supine
(page 99)

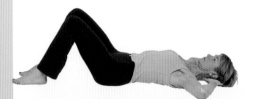

1 Lie on your back in neutral with knees bent. Place your hands under the back of your head with your elbows bent. **Inhale** to prepare.

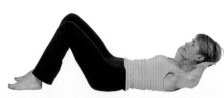

2 **Exhale**—float chest, neck, and head off the floor, keeping the weight of your head in your hands and neck and shoulders in alignment with your head. **Inhale** in this position. **Exhale**—lower chest, neck, and head.

Repeat 4–6 times.

Return to standing in neutral

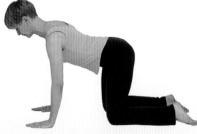

To end, relax by hugging the knees to the chest (see resting pose on page 112). Then roll onto your side and over onto all fours. Tuck your toes under and walk your hands toward your feet, shifting your weight back onto your feet. Keep your torso close to the ground.

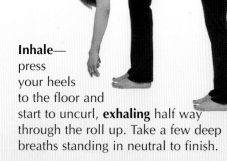

Inhale—press your heels to the floor and start to uncurl, **exhaling** half way through the roll up. Take a few deep breaths standing in neutral to finish.

Reaching a New Level

CHAPTER

About reaching a new level

Once you feel confident practicing the exercises from earlier chapters, especially the workout in Chapter 10, you are ready to take your Pilates further. These more advanced Pilates exercises require and build increased strength, mobility, and flexibility.

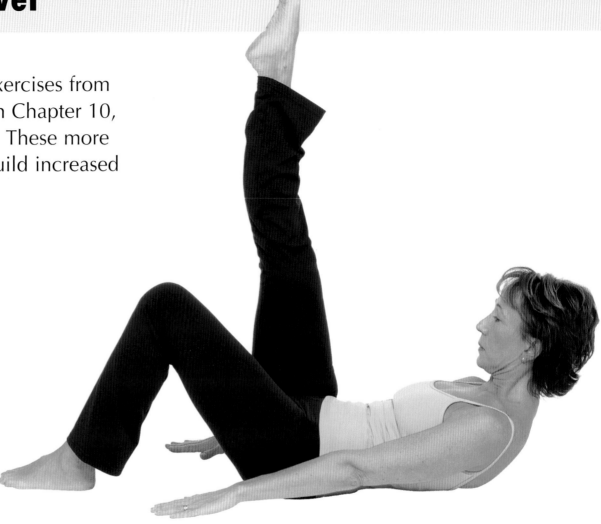

Practicing Pilates gives you a heightened awareness of your body and its needs. This awareness allows you to educate your muscles in a controlled but progressive way. That's the reason Pilates is often called "the thinking person's exercise."

Try these challenging exercises for a good test of your body awareness. If you have correctly practiced the movement and breathing coordination in the previous chapters, you should have discovered your body's strengths and weaknesses. If so, you will be able to select exercises in this chapter that you are ready to practice right away and recognize those you will need to work toward gradually.

As you do for all Pilates exercises, start by aligning yourself in neutral. For this workout, begin standing in neutral (see page 19). Once you have settled into a relaxed neutral position, practice your ribcage breathing before starting the Full Roll-Down warm-up.

The Full Roll-Down mobilizes and flexes your whole spine. It was covered in Chapter 4 but is featured again here as a warm-up. It is essential to stretch your spine before doing Pilates, especially when trying out exercises that make challenging demands on your muscles.

Visualization of the spine will help you to correctly coordinate your movements with your breathing. Imagine your spine as a string of pearls and that you are rolling up and down, one pearl at a time.

1 Stand in neutral with your feet hip-distance apart and your hips, knees, and ankles in alignment. **As you inhale,** slowly curl your head forward, followed by your neck and shoulders, and then roll down through the vertebrae of the upper back. As you go down, make sure your head, neck, shoulders, and arms are completely relaxed.

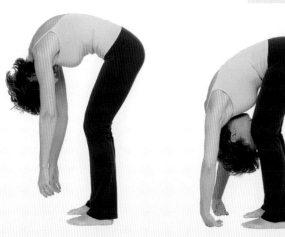

2 Continue rolling down, **exhaling as you pass waist level** and bending your knees slightly to take you down as far as you can go. Keep your knees, hips, and ankles in alignment so you are not sitting back into your hips.

3 **As you inhale,** start slowly uncurling. First drop your tailbone toward the floor, then uncurl through the lower back.

4 As your shoulders come up past your waist, **exhale** to uncurl through the upper back. Then bring your head up into alignment so you are back in neutral.

Repeat 4–6 times in a slow, flowing movement.

FORWARD FLEXION WITH LATERAL STRETCH

This challenging exercise focuses on bending forward and rotating the spine. If tight hamstrings prevent you from executing the movements accurately, you may want to come back to this one at a later date—once your continued practice of Pilates has loosened your hamstrings.

To get into position for the first step, follow steps 1 and 2 of the Full Roll-Down on page 117. When you have completed this exercise, exhale in the rolled-down position, then roll back up as in steps 3 and 4 on page 117.

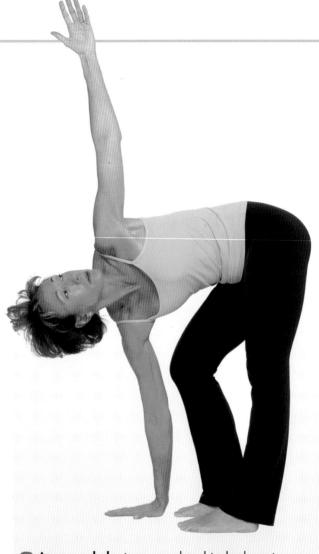

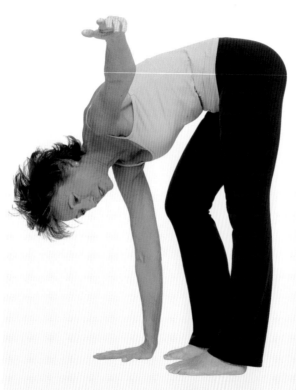

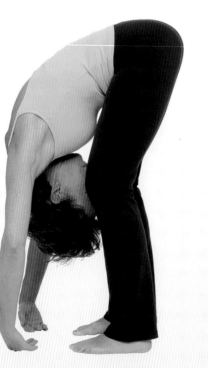

1 Stand in neutral. **As you inhale and then exhale,** slowly curl your head forward and roll all the way down as explained in steps 1 and 2 for the Full Roll-Down on page 117. Then place your hands flat on the floor.

2 **As you inhale,** extend your chest forward to maintain neutral pelvis, straighten your left leg, and slowly lift your left arm to the side and up toward the ceiling.

3 **As you exhale,** turn your head to look up to your left palm.
As you inhale, turn your head to look down.
As you exhale, lower your arm, head, neck, and chest back down, bending the left knee.

Repeat twice on each side alternately, following steps 2 and 3.

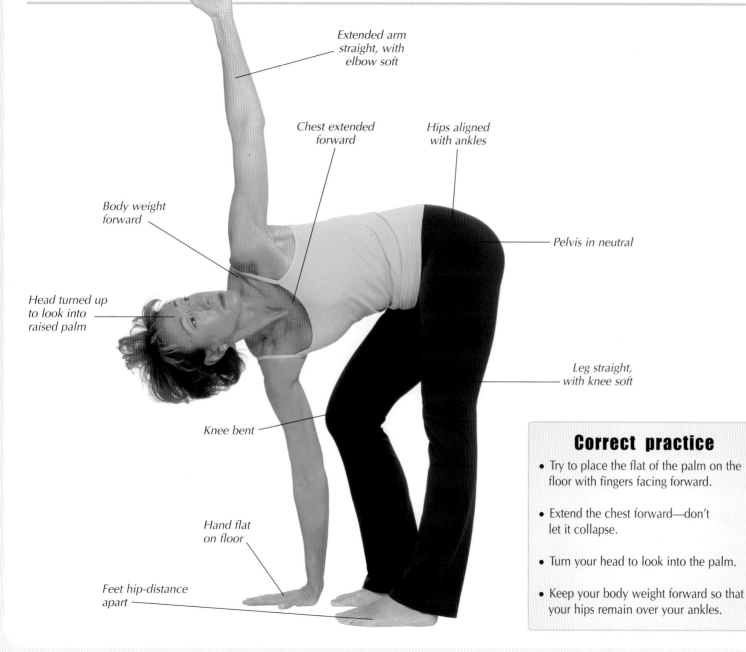

Extended arm straight, with elbow soft

Chest extended forward

Hips aligned with ankles

Body weight forward

Pelvis in neutral

Head turned up to look into raised palm

Leg straight, with knee soft

Knee bent

Hand flat on floor

Feet hip-distance apart

Make it easier

If you are not flexible enough to place your hands flat on the floor for this exercise, then touch the floor with your fingertips instead. You can also keep your knees bent if your hamstrings feel tight in this position. Always work within the range your flexibility allows.

Correct practice

- Try to place the flat of the palm on the floor with fingers facing forward.

- Extend the chest forward—don't let it collapse.

- Turn your head to look into the palm.

- Keep your body weight forward so that your hips remain over your ankles.

Focusing on balance and coordination, this exercise strengthens your calf muscles. You may find it difficult to maintain your balance at first, but with practice and the use of visualization you will quickly master this exercise.

1 Stand in neutral with your feet hip-distance apart and your hips, knees, and ankles in alignment.

Visualization

- As you rise onto your toes, imagine you are being lifted by a piece of string from the top of your head.

- Visualize your body like a rocket lifting off the ground in a perfectly straight line.

- Spread your toes as you rise onto the balls of your feet.

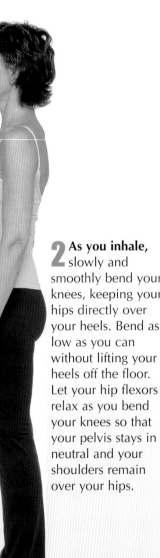

2 **As you inhale,** slowly and smoothly bend your knees, keeping your hips directly over your heels. Bend as low as you can without lifting your heels off the floor. Let your hip flexors relax as you bend your knees so that your pelvis stays in neutral and your shoulders remain over your hips.

3 **As you exhale,** slowly straighten your legs without completely locking your knee joints. As you straighten your legs, gently raise your heels off the floor and extend your tailbone down toward the floor, contracting the pelvic floor muscles and pulling the abdominal muscles inward and upward. Soften down through the front of your chest and keep your shoulders relaxed and over your hips.

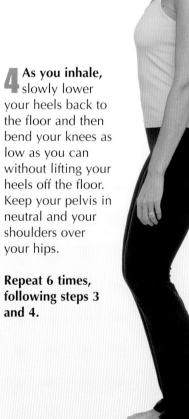

4 **As you inhale,** slowly lower your heels back to the floor and then bend your knees as low as you can without lifting your heels off the floor. Keep your pelvis in neutral and your shoulders over your hips.

Repeat 6 times, following steps 3 and 4.

KNEE BENDS WITH FORWARD FLEXION

This movement focuses on good posture and the correct alignment of the shoulders and hips as you extend forward. It works to strengthen the back muscles. By bending the knees and extending forward from the hip flexors, rather than the waist, this exercise, also known as Hip Hinging, will help to make you more aware of correct lifting and bending techniques.

1 Stand in neutral with your feet hip-distance apart and your hips, knees, and ankles in alignment.

2 As you inhale, gently bend your knees, keeping your hips directly over your heels. Go as low as you can without lifting your heels off the floor. Let your hip flexors relax as you bend your knees so that your pelvis stays in neutral and your shoulders remain over your hips.

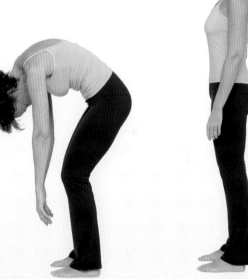

3 As you exhale, slowly extend your torso forward from your hips using your hip flexors. Extend your tailbone back and bring your shoulders level with your hips. Reach your arms along the sides of your body to draw your shoulders away from your head. Keep the top of your head extending forward. Lengthen through your torso with your chest extending forward.

4 As you inhale, slowly fold your torso over your bent knees without shifting your body weight backward. Let your head, neck, shoulders, and arms relax completely.

5 As you exhale, gently uncurl your spine, drawing your abdominal muscles in and engaging your pelvic floor muscles. Keep your shoulders relaxed and finish in neutral, ready to repeat.

Repeat 4–6 times in a smooth, continuous movement.

KNEE BEND WITH FORWARD FLEXION IN FOCUS

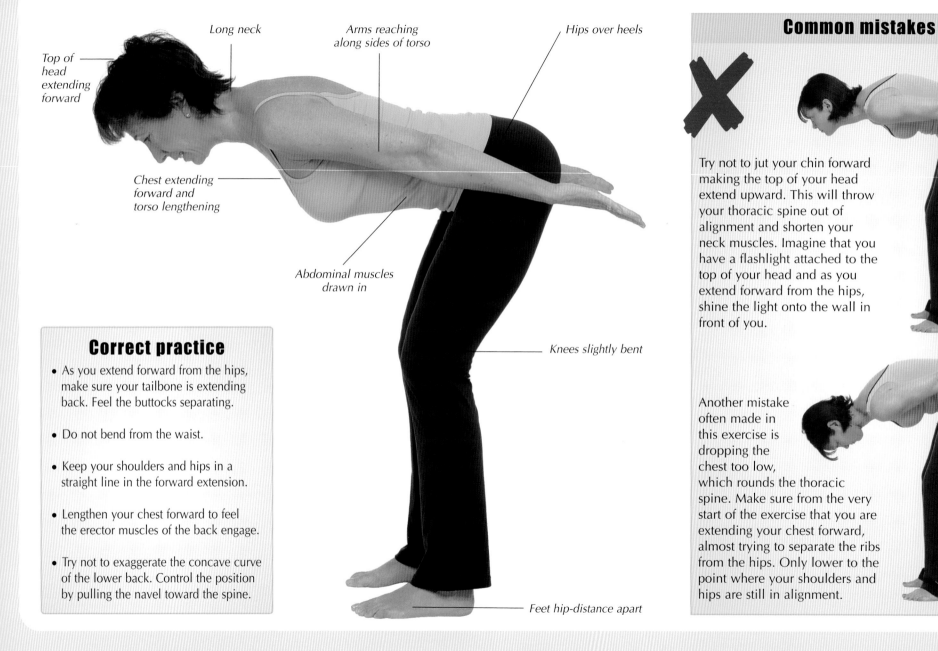

Top of head extending forward

Long neck

Arms reaching along sides of torso

Hips over heels

Chest extending forward and torso lengthening

Abdominal muscles drawn in

Knees slightly bent

Feet hip-distance apart

Correct practice

- As you extend forward from the hips, make sure your tailbone is extending back. Feel the buttocks separating.

- Do not bend from the waist.

- Keep your shoulders and hips in a straight line in the forward extension.

- Lengthen your chest forward to feel the erector muscles of the back engage.

- Try not to exaggerate the concave curve of the lower back. Control the position by pulling the navel toward the spine.

Common mistakes

Try not to jut your chin forward making the top of your head extend upward. This will throw your thoracic spine out of alignment and shorten your neck muscles. Imagine that you have a flashlight attached to the top of your head and as you extend forward from the hips, shine the light onto the wall in front of you.

Another mistake often made in this exercise is dropping the chest too low, which rounds the thoracic spine. Make sure from the very start of the exercise that you are extending your chest forward, almost trying to separate the ribs from the hips. Only lower to the point where your shoulders and hips are still in alignment.

PLIÉS WITH LATERAL STRETCH

This exercise focuses on coordination and lengthening the lateral muscles while keeping the pelvis in neutral.

1 Stand in neutral with your feet hip-distance apart and your hips, knees, and ankles in alignment. Move your legs apart to a wide but comfortable position. Turn your feet out as far as you can while still keeping your kneecaps in line with your toes.

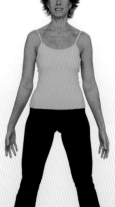

2 **As you inhale,** gently bend your knees and slowly float your arms up to shoulder height.

3 **As you exhale,** slowly lift your right arm up toward the ceiling and tilt your torso to the left. Keep your hips facing forward and level, and lengthen the ribs up and over to the side from the waist. As the torso bends, let your head tilt as well.

4 **As you inhale,** slowly return to the center with your arms extending to the sides at shoulder height.

5 **As you exhale,** gently lift your left arm up toward the ceiling and tilt your torso to the right. Keep your hips facing forward and level and lengthen the ribs up and over to the side from the waist. As the torso bends, let your head tilt as well.

6 **As you inhale,** slowly return to the center with your arms extending to the sides at shoulder height.

Repeat 4–6 times on each side alternately, in a continuous movement.

SEATED SPINAL ROTATION WITH FORWARD FLEXION

This multi-joint movement is challenging. You need strong hip flexors and core stability muscles as you sit up over your hips while rotating the torso, keeping the pelvis in neutral and the hamstrings lengthening. As you become more flexible, you will enjoy the sensation of this exercise and the sense of achievement. It should be performed in a fluid and continuous movement.

1 Sit in neutral with your legs at least shoulder-width apart, fully extended along the floor. Extend your arms out to your sides at shoulder height and relax your shoulders.

2 **As you inhale,** gently rotate your shoulders and torso from the waist to the left, keeping both buttocks imprinting into the floor. Keep your arms relaxed and still as your body twists.

3 **As you exhale,** slowly reach your right arm toward your left foot. As you move, pull your abdominal muscles in toward the spine. Keep both buttocks on the floor, shoulders relaxed, and left arm extending behind.

4 **As you inhale,** gently lift your torso back to the rotated position.

5 **As you exhale,** slowly rotate your torso back to the center position.

Repeat 4–6 times on each side alternately, in a smooth, continuous movement.

As you rotate...

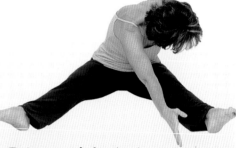

- As you rotate, keep your spine lengthening and your pelvis in neutral. Keep both sitz bones imprinting into the floor.

- If you find it hard to keep your shoulders down and relaxed, try turning your palms to the ceiling.

- Carry your arms with the shoulder girdle and do not push them beyond their range of movement.

- Follow the back hand with your focus.

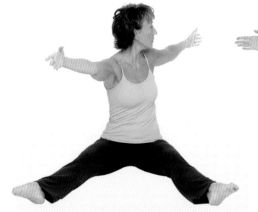
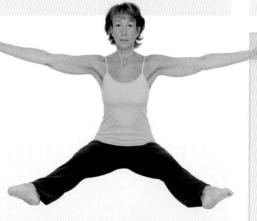
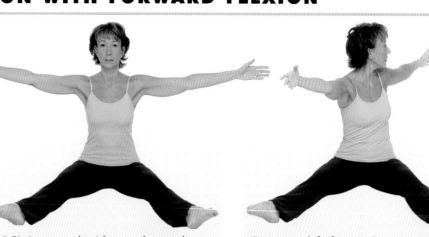

FULL ROLL-DOWN FROM SEATED POSITION

This multi-task exercise lengthens and strengthens the back and abdominal muscles and is extremely challenging. You need strong abdominal muscles, a well-balanced posture, and long hamstrings to execute it well. You may find it impossible to perform at first, and it will require patience and practice to master. Do the Bridge exercise in Chapter 5 and the deep abdominal exercises in Chapter 9 to prepare yourself.

Correct practice

- Perform this exercise slowly and with control.

- Maintain the deep abdominal contraction as you exhale.

- Lengthen through your legs as you roll down and up. Do not allow your shoulders to hunch and lift when rolling up; keep them relaxed.

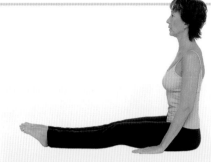

1 Sit in neutral with your legs fully extended along the floor. Extend your arms forward above the thighs at chest level and relax your shoulders.

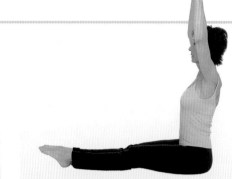

2 **As you inhale,** gently lift your arms above your head, keeping your shoulders down and lengthening through your torso.

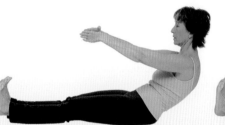

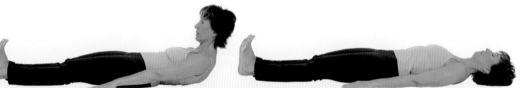

3 **As you exhale,** contract deeply through the abdominals, closing the front of the ribcage and engaging the pelvic floor muscles. Flex your feet and slowly roll down through the spine. Imprint each vertebra into the floor as you roll down.

Allow your arms to draw down to your sides and place your fingertips on the floor as you are rolling down. Finish with the whole length of your body and your head on the floor.

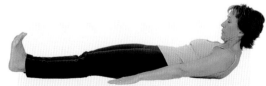

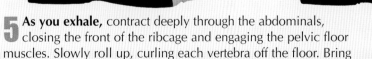

4 **As you inhale,** slowly curl your head, neck, and shoulders off the floor, focusing on your toes.

5 **As you exhale,** contract deeply through the abdominals, closing the front of the ribcage and engaging the pelvic floor muscles. Slowly roll up, curling each vertebra off the floor. Bring your arms back up and point your feet. **Inhale** in this position.

Repeat steps 3 to 5 four to six times. Exhale and lower arms.

SCISSORS

Scissors is similar to Single Leg Extensions on page 101, but the legs are kept lengthened as they move up and down. Fully extended legs create more body resistance and increase the challenge to the core stability muscles. The main objective of the exercise is to keep the abdominals as flat as possible while performing the exercise and to work each side of the abdominals separately.

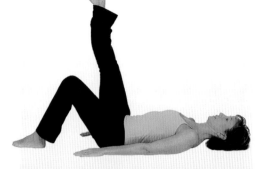

1 Lie on your back in neutral with knees bent, arms at your sides, and ankles and knees hip-distance apart. Extend one leg toward the ceiling, keeping ankle, knee, and hip in alignment. Keep your pelvis in neutral and the other knee bent with the foot on the floor. **Inhale** to prepare.

2 **As you exhale,** slowly curl your head, neck, and chest up. Keeping your fingertips on the floor, reach your arms along the floor, relaxing and drawing your shoulders away from your neck.

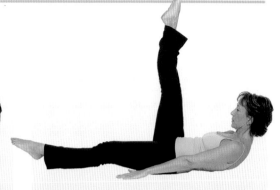

3 **As you inhale,** keep the lifted leg in position and extend the other leg along the floor.

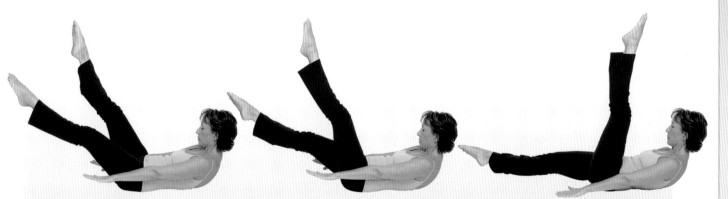

4 **As you exhale,** keep your chest in the cervical curl position and alternate your leg positions, lowering the upper leg to the floor while simultaneously lifting the lower leg to the vertical position. Keep pulling in the abdominal muscles as the legs swap position.

Blow the air out of your lungs quite vigorously **on the exhale** and then take a very small **inhale.**

Repeat the scissor movement 10–12 times as in step 4.

Correct practice

- As you repeat the scissors movement, keep the chest in the cervical curl position and shoulders down.

- Change the leg positions so that the upper leg lowers to the floor and the lower leg lifts to the vertical position at the same time. Keep pulling the abdominal muscles in as the legs change position. Always bring the legs to the position shown in step 3 as you swap them. Keep lengthening the legs.

- Blow the air out quite vigorously **on the exhale** as the leg positions swap and take a very small **inhale.** It should feel like you are blowing out lots of candles on a cake.

- Retain a neutral spine throughout the exercise.

This exercise challenges the abdominal muscles while the arms and legs are extended. It helps to improve mobility of the shoulder joints and coordination of your deep breathing with arm and leg movements. As it requires strength and control of all the muscles of the torso, it should only be performed a maximum of four times at this level, with a half a second rest between each repetition.

CAUTION: If you have a weak back, do not attempt this exercise.

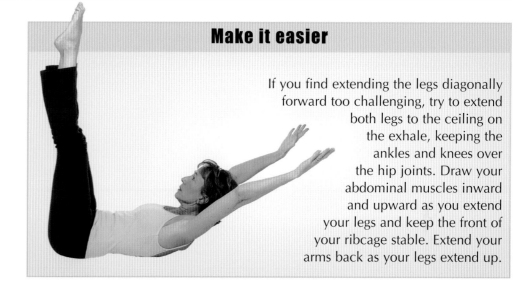

Make it easier

If you find extending the legs diagonally forward too challenging, try to extend both legs to the ceiling on the exhale, keeping the ankles and knees over the hip joints. Draw your abdominal muscles inward and upward as you extend your legs and keep the front of your ribcage stable. Extend your arms back as your legs extend up.

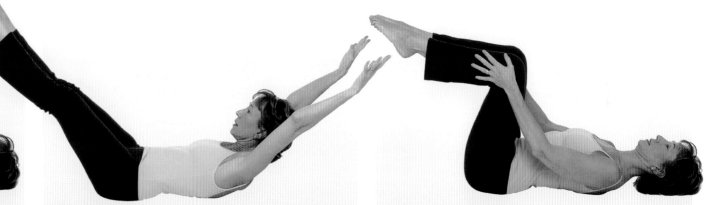

1 Lie in neutral with your head, neck, and shoulders resting on the floor and your arms at your sides on the floor. Float one knee at a time to a right-angle position so that your knees are bent and directly over your hips and your ankles form a straight horizontal line with your knees. Rest your hands on the sides of your knees. **As you inhale,** draw your chin down toward your neck without tensing your shoulders.

2 **As you exhale,** slowly extend both legs forward diagonally from the hips. At the same time, curl your head, neck, shoulders, and chest off the floor and extend both arms back as far as possible, drawing your abdominal muscles inward and upward as you extend the legs and arms and keeping the front of the ribcage stable.

3 **As you inhale,** slowly return to the starting position.

Repeat 4 times in a slow, continuous movement.

SWAN DIVE—PRONE

This is another exercise for strengthening the upper back muscles while stabilizing the torso. The Swan Dive also helps to improve the strength and mobility in your back.

1 Lie face down in neutral. Place the tip of your nose on the floor and your palms on the floor at your sides, at shoulder level. Keep your pelvis in neutral and your legs extending along the floor. **Inhale** slowly to prepare.

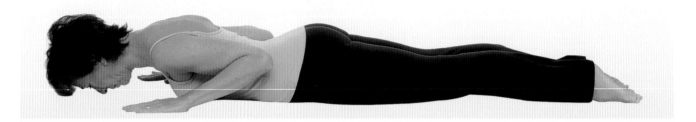

2 **As you exhale,** draw your abdominal muscles in, draw your shoulders away from your ears, and float your head, neck, and chest off the floor. Extend your breastbone forward as you lift. Engage your pelvic floor muscles to keep your pelvis in its neutral position.

Upper back flexibility

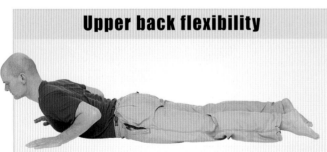

If your upper back is very flexible, it will look like this when you do the Swan Dive. Aim for the greatest flexibility your body will allow.

3 **As you inhale,** slowly lower your chest back down and lift your legs off the floor while keeping your pubic bone and hipbones on the floor.

Repeat 4–6 times in a slow, continuous movement.

OPPOSITE ARM AND LEG EXTENSIONS

This is an excellent exercise for strengthening the back and abdominal muscles, streamlining the hips and buttocks, and improving awareness of your technique and coordination skills.

Correct practice

Make sure the arm and leg work in unison with your breathing and that when they are moving your torso is still and your spine remains in neutral.

1 Start on all fours in neutral with your joints in alignment. **As you inhale,** extend your right arm and left leg along the floor to prepare for the first lift.

2 **As you exhale,** slowly lift your extended arm and leg to shoulder and hip height. Draw your abdominal muscles up toward the spine.

3 **As you inhale,** lower your arm and leg back down to the starting position.

Repeat the lifts 4–6 times on this side.

4 **As you exhale,** move back into your neutral all fours position.
As you inhale, extend your left arm and your right leg along the floor to prepare for the right leg lift.

5 **As you exhale,** lift your extended arm and leg to shoulder and hip height.
As you inhale, lower your arm and leg.

Repeat the lifts 4–6 times on this side.

Prayer Stretch

During a strenuous exercise routine, use this resting pose to gently stretch the front of the shoulders and the back, pectoral, and quadraceps muscles. From a kneeling position, bring your buttocks down onto your heels. Rest your forehead on the floor and extend your arms in front of you. **Inhale** and **exhale** deeply to gently stretch and relax your spine.

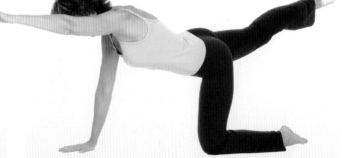

This 12–15-minute routine is more advanced than the workout in Chapter 10, so make sure that you have mastered the individual exercises before trying it out. Leave out the Leg and Arm Extensions from Right Angle if you have a weak back.

Once you have been doing this routine for a while and feel ready to move to an even higher level, add Scissors (page 126) after the Full Roll-Down from Seated Position.

Stand in neutral and do some deep ribcage breathing practice before starting the Full Roll-Down for your warm-up. Keep the movements flowing and move in time with your breathing.

Full Roll-Down
(page 117)

1 Inhale—start to roll down.

2 Exhale—roll all the way down.
Inhale and exhale—roll back up.

Repeat 4 times.

Forward Flexion with Lateral Stretch (page 118)

1 Inhale—from rolled-down position, straighten left leg and float up left arm.

2 Exhale—turn head up.
Inhale—turn head down.
Exhale—lower arm.

Repeat twice on each side alternately.

Knee Bends with Heel Raise
(page 120)

1 Inhale—lower with heels on floor.

2 Exhale—rise onto toes.

Repeat 6 times.

Knee Bends with Forward Flexion (page 121)

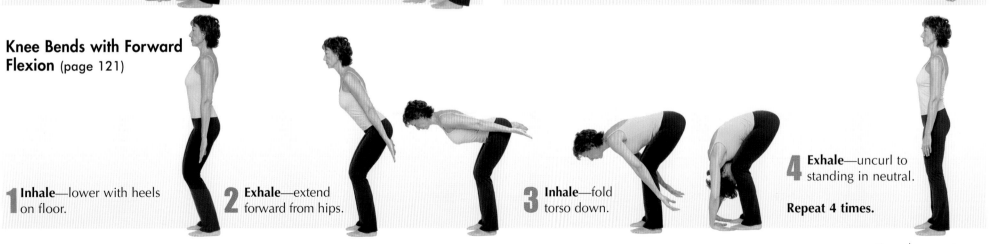

1 Inhale—lower with heels on floor.

2 Exhale—extend forward from hips.

3 Inhale—fold torso down.

4 Exhale—uncurl to standing in neutral.

Repeat 4 times.

continued on next page

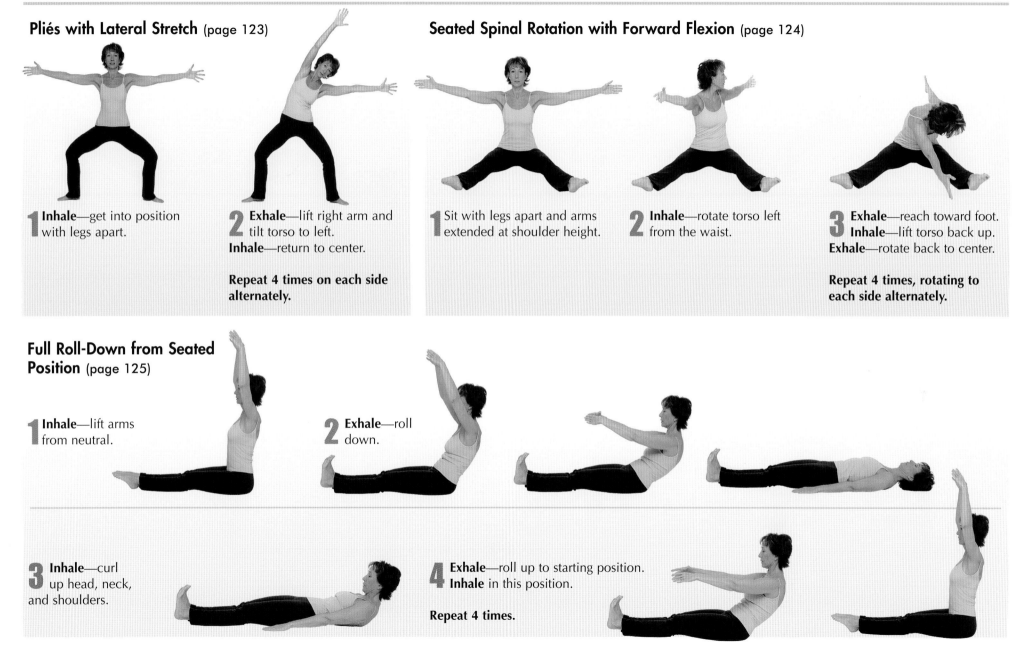

Pliés with Lateral Stretch (page 123)

1 Inhale—get into position with legs apart.

2 Exhale—lift right arm and tilt torso to left.
Inhale—return to center.

Repeat 4 times on each side alternately.

Seated Spinal Rotation with Forward Flexion (page 124)

1 Sit with legs apart and arms extended at shoulder height.

2 Inhale—rotate torso left from the waist.

3 Exhale—reach toward foot.
Inhale—lift torso back up.
Exhale—rotate back to center.

Repeat 4 times, rotating to each side alternately.

Full Roll-Down from Seated Position (page 125)

1 Inhale—lift arms from neutral.

2 Exhale—roll down.

3 Inhale—curl up head, neck, and shoulders.

4 Exhale—roll up to starting position.
Inhale in this position.

Repeat 4 times.

continued on next page

Leg and Arm Extensions from Right Angle
(page 127)

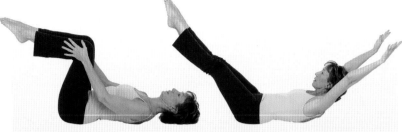

1 Start with legs at right angle and hands on knees.
Inhale—draw chin down toward neck.

2 **Exhale**—extend legs and arms and curl up.
Inhale—return to starting position.

Repeat 4 times.

Swan Dive—Prone (page 128)

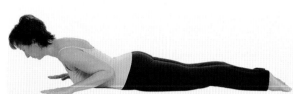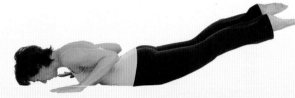

1 **Inhale** to prepare, lying in neutral with palms on floor at shoulder height.
Exhale—float head, neck, and chest up.

2 **Inhale**—lower chest and lift legs.

Repeat 4 times.

Opposite Arm and Leg Extensions (page 129)

1 **Inhale**—extend right arm and left leg.

2 **Exhale**—lift arm and leg.

3 **Inhale**—lower arm and leg.

**Lift and lower 4 times.
Repeat on other side.**

Finish standing in neutral

1 Come back into the all fours position and tuck the toes under.
Inhale to prepare.

2 **Exhale**—lift your knees off the floor, straightening the legs and extending the tailbone upward to create a pyramid shape. Keep your palms on the floor and walk your feet in to your hands, bending your knees.

3 **Inhale**—slowly uncurl your torso. As your head passes your waist, start **exhaling** and uncurl to an upright position.

Take a couple of deep breaths in a good posture before finishing.

12

Pilates for Healing

Pilates for healing

Physical therapists and osteopaths often recommend Pilates exercises to both relieve and prevent muscular tensions, aches, and pains. This chapter features Pilates exercises that you can practice for self-help.

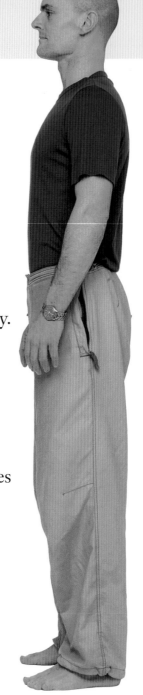

Contemporary lifestyles mean that people need to spend more time and effort undoing bad postural habits than ever before. Many aches and pains are caused by muscular weakness and imbalances. For example, tight muscles in the legs and lower back can cause lower-back pain and poor posture. Pilates exercises will help to remedy these imbalances and relieve discomfort, but learning to use your body correctly can minimize injury in the first place.

In this chapter the author works with an osteopathic physician to provide valuable advice on how to lift and carry correctly to prevent injury. She also gives exercises specially designed to relieve chronic muscle pains and stiffness in the back.

But remember, if you experience pain in your back or joints, always consult your doctor before starting any exercise regime. Pilates exercises are low impact and are performed within your range of flexibility, so they will not put undue strain on joints or muscles. With continued exercise you will gradually and gently strengthen your body, easing away many minor aches and pains that you thought were inevitable!

Tips for a healthy spine

- Regularly check your posture in the mirror (see page 18). Rounded shoulders and a jutting chin could indicate that you are spending too much time leaning over a desk at work. Try to improve your seated posture (see page 85).

- Use a backrest or a lumbar roll for support when sitting for very long periods. Get up and move around often to prevent your lumbar spine from stiffening up.

- Don't put up with back pain. Consult a doctor, physical therapist, or osteopathic physician to find the cause of the problem. Lower-back pain is not caused by drafts, chills, or the weather.

- Maintain good posture when practicing all activities and sports.

- Practice Pilates at least once a week to help strengthen your core stability muscles and back. It will make you more aware of how to use your body more efficiently.

Back pain, especially in the lower back, is often the result of bad posture. Sitting for long periods, repeated bending, heavy lifting, and standing or lying in awkward positions can all create back pain. If this rings a bell with you, then take steps to improve your posture when lifting, sitting, and carrying.

How to lift items correctly

Your lifestyle or job may not involve lots of lifting, but it takes only one mistake to injure your spine. Whenever you have to lift a heavy object, make sure you keep your spine in alignment. If the object is on the floor, first lower yourself on bended knees. Then, keeping your back straight, lift by using the power of your legs. This avoids putting stress on your spine that could injure your back.

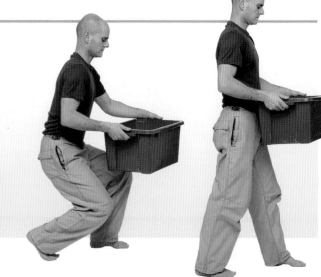

Seated exercise to mobilize the spine

If you are unable to get up and move about for long periods, perhaps during a plane or car journey or while sitting in the office, practice this simple exercise at least once every hour. It increases the blood supply to your spine and stops the joints from becoming fixed in one position.

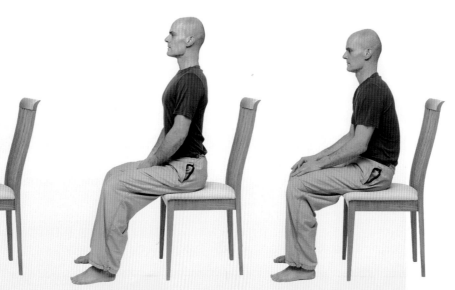

1 Sit forward in your seat with your spine aligned.

2 Keeping your neck and shoulders still, tilt your pelvis forward, exaggerating the curve of your lumbar spine, then backward, rounding your back.

Repeat for about 5 minutes once every hour.

Carrying in alignment

It's hard to go anywhere today without having to carry a bag of essentials, whether it's for work, study, or domestic errands. When carrying a bag, always maintain a stable, upright posture. Make sure you alternate the shoulder or arm you use to carry the weight to prevent an imbalance of strength and spinal alignment.

This exercise stretches the muscles of the hips and lower back. It is a good exercise for both relieving and preventing the muscle tension that causes lower-back pain. Start with several knee sways to gently mobilize your hips, lower back, and pelvic joints and then stretch the leg on the last knee sway.

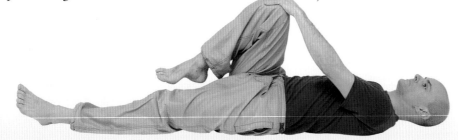

1 Lie on your back in neutral. Extend your right arm out to the side and bend your right knee, lengthening the left leg along the floor. Hold your bent knee with your left hand. **Inhale** in this position, trying to maintain neutral spine.

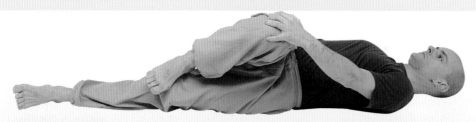

2 As you exhale, gently pull your right knee over to the left side with your left hand, keeping the right shoulder on the floor.

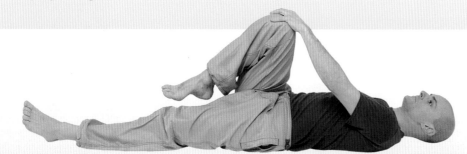

3 As you inhale, bring your knee back to the starting position.

Repeat steps 2 and 3 eight times, bringing the knee closer to the floor each time.

4 As you exhale, gently pull your right knee over again and this time extend your leg along the floor.

5 As you inhale, bring your knee back to the starting position.

Repeat with the left leg and right arm.

Alternative exercise for lower-back relief

The Pelvic Rock (see page 47) is another good Pilates exercise for easing and alleviating lower-back tension, and it is a gentler exercise than the Leg Crossover. If you find it more comfortable to lie on your front, do the Pelvic Tilt instead (see page 63).

Tight hamstrings can cause hip-joint problems, which can, in turn, lead to lower-back pain. So when practicing Pilates to relieve or prevent lower-back pain, include this Hamstring Lengthener in your routine. It is also a good exercise for stretching the muscles of the spine, the hips, and the calves and relieving tension in those areas.

Start this exercise by rolling down following steps 1 and 2 of the Full Roll-Down (see page 39). At the end of the exercise, roll up following steps 3 and 4 of the Full Roll-Down. You may find it more comfortable when rolling down to bend forward from the hips until you reach waist level, as seen on page 121, then drop the head and gently roll the spine down the rest of the way.

If you cannot touch your hands to the floor for this exercise, bend your knees. Or if you prefer to stretch your hamstrings while lying on your back, turn to page 58.

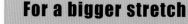

For a bigger stretch

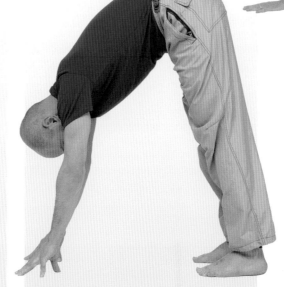

Everyone has their own range of flexibility. You may be very flexible in some joints and not in others. If it's within your range of movement, walk your hands out farther when doing the Hamstring Lengthener than step 3 shows.

When your arms are in a position that forms a straight line with your back (a pyramid shape), place your hands flat on the floor. Hold for 15 seconds, **inhaling** and **exhaling**, and then walk your hands back in.

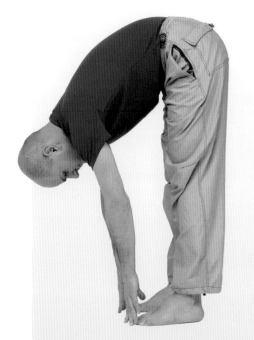

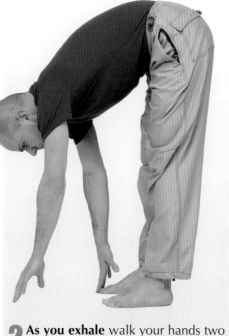

1 Stand in your neutral spine position and roll your torso down, **inhaling** and **exhaling** as you roll down. **Inhale** in the rolled down position.

2 **As you exhale** walk your hands two paces forward, keeping your legs straight.

3 Hold for 15 seconds, **inhaling** and **exhaling**, then walk your hands back in and roll back up to the standing position.

The aim here is to relieve back tension, especially in the upper back (the thoracic region). You can also practice it as a preventive exercise to improve the flexibility of your upper back and neck (the thoracic and cervical spine), where the movement of the spine is often restricted by weak, tight muscles.

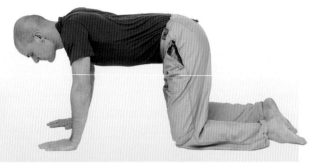

1 Kneel on all fours in neutral and check your Pilates alignment. **Inhale** in this neutral position to prepare.

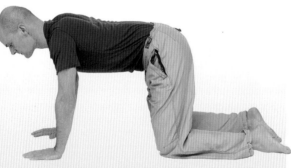

2 **As you exhale,** slowly draw your shoulder blades together and, at the same time, raise your head slightly. Keep your pelvis in neutral, moving only your upper spine, shoulder blades, and neck.

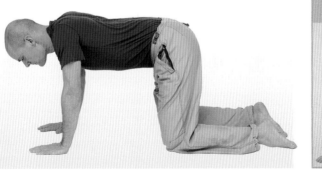

3 **As you inhale,** slowly return your shoulder blades, spine, and neck to the neutral position.

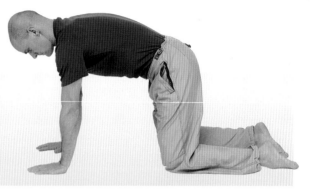

4 **As you exhale,** slowly draw your shoulder blades apart and at the same time drop your head slightly. Keep your pelvis in neutral, moving only your upper spine, shoulder blades, and neck.

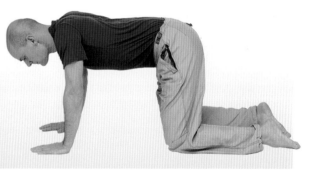

5 **As you inhale,** slowly return your shoulder blades, spine, and neck to the neutral position.

Repeat 4–6 times.

Alternative general back relief

The Bridge is another good exercise to practice when your back is feeling uncomfortable (see page 49). Pilates exercises that involve rotation or sideways stretches can also help relieve tension in the back. These include the Lateral Stretch, Knee Sways, and Seated Spinal Rotation with Forward Flexion (see pages 41, 51, and 124).

Here are exercises to help relieve shoulder and neck tension. The Pectoral Stretch focuses on opening the chest and stretching the pectoral muscles, which, if tight, cause the shoulders to become rounded.

The Shoulder Stretch and Arm Cross are exercises you can do to loosen shoulder tension at work or on long journeys.

Shoulder Stretch

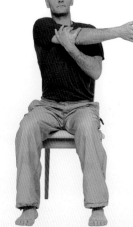

Sit with your buttocks and back against the chair back, your shoulders over your hips and your legs hip-distance apart. Extend your right arm across your chest and hold it with your left hand just above the elbow.
Inhale, keeping the shoulder relaxed.
As you exhale, gently increase the stretch by pressing your right elbow closer to your chest.

Repeat twice on each arm alternately.

Pectoral Stretch

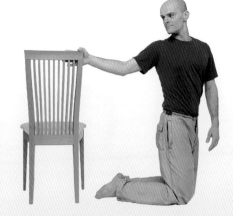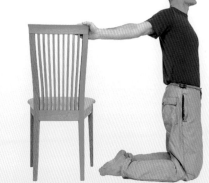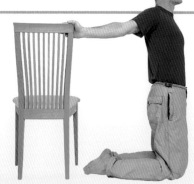

1 Kneel with your knees and ankles together, an arms-length away from a chair as shown. Place one hand on the top of the chair back.

2 **As you inhale,** slowly rotate your torso from the waist to look at the chair. Keep your hips facing forward.

3 **As you exhale,** rotate your torso away from the chair, extending your arm and bringing your shoulders back into alignment with your hips. Keep your shoulders down and relaxed. You should feel the stretch across the front of the chest and in the shoulder area.

Repeat 2–3 times on each side.

Arm Cross

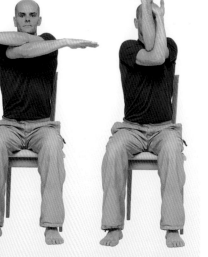

1 Sit in neutral. **As you inhale,** lift both arms in front of your chest and cross them at the elbow.

2 **As you exhale,** lift your forearms upward, then intertwine the hand of the lower arm around the top arm with palms toward each other and thumbs toward you. Hold this position, **inhaling** and **exhaling** to stretch the upper back and shoulder muscles.

Swap the arms over and repeat.

Relieving headaches

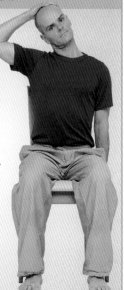

If you have a persistent headache, it could be caused by tight, sore neck muscles. Before you resort to medication, try this exercise.

Sit on a straight-back chair, holding the edge of the chair with your left hand. Place your right hand on top of your head. **Inhale** in this position. **As you exhale,** tilt your head to the right, lengthening your neck muscles. Apply minimal pressure with your hand. Hold for 15 seconds, breathing deeply.

Repeat 6 times, alternating sides.

The models in this book have all studied Pilates for a few years or more. Many now teach the skills they have learned. All enjoy improved strength and flexibility as a result of their Pilates workouts.

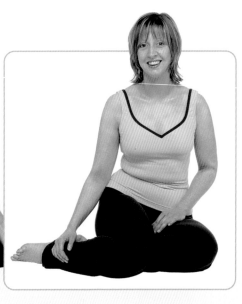

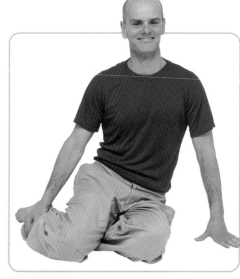

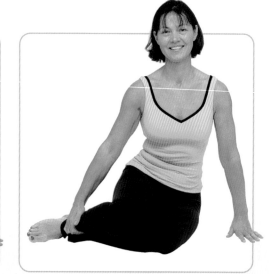

Carolan Brown is a trained choreographer and dancer and a certified Pilates and aerobics instructor. She has been a fitness instructor for over 20 years and achieved celebrity when she became personal trainer to Diana, The Princess of Wales. Carolan has produced exercise videos, advised on health and fitness on TV and radio in the United Kingdom and Canada, and been featured in women's magazines in Britain and the United States. She currently works as a Pilates teacher and personal trainer at her studio—the Soma Centre—in Richmond upon Thames, Surrey. Her holistic center is dedicated to improving and maintaining total fitness. Married with two children, Carolan lives in London.

Sarah Collyer, 34, is a market research director. A regular Pilates student, she came to Pilates just over three years ago following an illness. Unable to continue attending the gym, she was looking for a physical activity that was calming and wouldn't put her body under strain. Pilates appealed to her because of its similarity to ballet, which she had studied for 10 years as an adolescent and teenager. Sarah feels that practicing Pilates has been enormously beneficial to her, both physically and mentally. Her figure has changed shape, and her hips and legs have slimmed down. Mentally, she feels "in balance" and more aware of her body during her everyday life. This year she broke two ribs and is convinced that her Pilates exercise helped her to recover more quickly.

Luis Illueca, 39, started out as a sports masseur and fitness instructor and is now an osteopath naturopath. He has practiced Pilates for nearly four years and does biomechanical assessments for Pilates students at Carolan's Soma Centre— watching students walk and move in their classes, he points out pelvic or musculature imbalances that they need to focus on with their exercises. Luis was drawn to Pilates because of its scientific approach, which fits in well with how he approaches the body when practicing osteopathy. Because his job is physically strenuous, he needs to keep fit. Though swimming is his main form of exercise, he considers his weekly Pilates exercises essential for maintaining a strong and flexible spine.

Mandy Mitchell, 45, is a cabin service director with British Airways. She has been practicing Pilates for seven years and was certified as an instructor by the Physical Mind Institute, New York. Her interest in Pilates started only after she had been teaching fitness for 10 years. It appealed to her because she felt it offered functional exercises using breathing techniques in conjunction with movements that both lengthened and strengthened the muscles without putting any weight or strain on the joints. Mandy feels that Pilates helps keep her postural muscles strong and alleviates any back pain suffered from her physically demanding job and her other activities, which include horseback riding, jumping horses, and showing dogs.

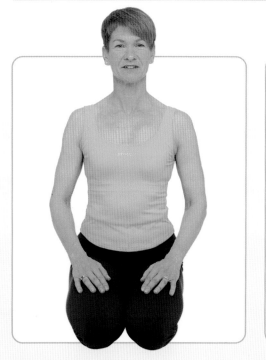 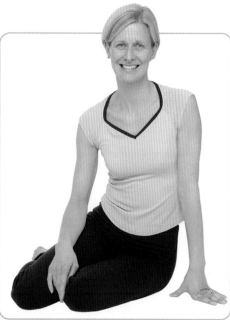 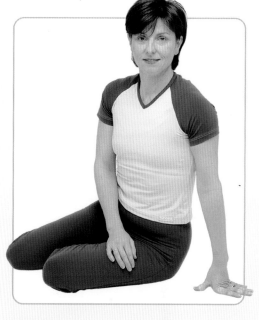 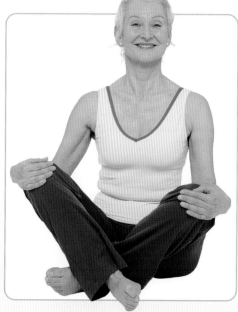

Rosemary Newman is a full-time Pilates and fitness instructor, as well as a mother of two boys, aged 18 and 22. She has been practicing Pilates for about four years, ever since she heard how good it is for strengthening the back and abdominals and for improving posture. As a reformed "sloucher," Rosemary says that Pilates has helped her realign her body and "stand tall." Her students include men and women of all ages and abilities, including those with back problems, and pre- and post-natal women. Rosemary finds that Pilates builds her students' self-confidence. It has also relieved many of back and neck discomfort and headaches. One of her students even become free of tinnitus after suffering for eight years.

Sarah Riglin, 38, is a full-time mother to three children and a part-time student of Pilates. She became interested in Pilates while she was experiencing back problems during pregnancy, having heard that it is good for realigning your body. She has studied Pilates for two years and feels that she has really progressed in that time, that her posture has improved, and that she generally looks fitter. As a busy mother, Sarah can only fit in a Pilates class once a week and looks forward to having more time for this when her children are older.

Mary Store is a Pilates instructor and a mother of three. Following the birth of her third child nine years ago and the subsequent shedding of 70 pounds, she qualified as a group exercise instructor. Four years ago she attended her first Pilates class and was instantly hooked and inspired. Twelve months later she qualified as a Pilates instructor. Although she has become a dramatically stronger, longer, and leaner individual through Pilates, she gets even more satisfaction from hearing her students relate their own significant improvements in strength, postural awareness, and overall well-being. Mary believes that practicing Pilates is a lifestyle change and that all its benefits are carried over to everyday life.

Nina Taunton is a lecturer in Shakespeare and Renaissance Studies at Brunel University in London and a student of Pilates. She came to Pilates, studying with Carolan Brown, late in life but now says she would "rather cut off a toe than miss a class." In her job, Nina sits for hours at a time, reading, writing, and working at her computer. Pilates helps avert potential problems here; it loosens shoulder tension and alleviates back strain. It has also increased her flexibility and has contributed to an almost complete recovery of movement, suppleness, and strength in an arm very badly broken six years ago.

GLOSSARY

ALIGNMENT
In this position your spine retains its natural curves, your pelvis is in neutral, your shoulders are level, your head and neck are relaxed, with the back of your neck extending, and your gaze faces forward. You minimize your body's structural imbalances and your posture is straight.

BALANCE
When your spine is in neutral and each side of your body carries an equal amount of body weight, and your muscles are able to support your joints, you have muscular balance. If your spine is misaligned, your muscles compensate, creating an imbalance.

CERVICAL
A term that relates to the vertebrae of the neck. There are five cervical vertebrae. The first connects the base of your skull to your spine.

CORE MUSCLES
Responsible for good posture, these are the abdominal, back, and pelvic floor muscles which are all attached to the spine. For core stability these muscles need to be engaged.

ENGAGING THE MUSCLES
To create a strong center and hold your torso in neutral, your pelvic floor and abdominal muscles need to be tightened. To do this, draw up the muscles of the pelvic floor and hollow the abdominal muscles back

toward your spine as you exhale. It is important not to overtighten or clench your muscles, however.

EXTEND
This is achieved when you stretch a limb so that it moves away from the body, such as raising your arms above your head.

FLEX
This is achieved when you bend a limb so that it moves closer to the body, such as raising your knee so the upper part of your leg moves toward you.

IMPRINTING
This is achieved when you press your bones into the floor and can feel them making contact with the floor. This will make you aware of being in correct alignment. For example, when sitting in neutral you should feel your sitz bones pressing into the floor, and be aware of a slight muscular tension around the bones that are imprinting.

KYPHOSIS
An abnormal curvature of the upper spine that creates round shoulders and a hump back. The curvature can affect the neck, making the chin poke forward. People with round shoulders often have tight neck and chest muscles, too.

LOCKED
When a joint such as the knee or elbow is overextended, it is locked.

LORDOSIS
The hollow in the lower back (also called the lumbar curve). The depth of the natural curve varies from person to person but the term is more often used to indicate an exaggerated lumbar curve.

LUMBAR
A term that relates to the five vertebrae of the lower back. These massive weight-bearing vertebrae have limited movement. The lumbar vertebrae link to the thoracic vertebrae of the upper back and the sacrum, which forms part of the pelvic girdle.

NEUTRAL PELVIS
Your pelvis is said to be in neutral when it is correctly aligned, your tailbone is extending to the floor, and your buttocks are relaxed. This position helps you retain the natural curves of the spine and good muscle balance.

NEUTRAL SPINE
When your major joints—the ankles, knees, hips, and shoulders—are aligned and the natural curvature of your spine is retained, your spine is in its neutral position.

PELVIC FLOOR MUSCLES
Spanning the inside of the pelvis, these muscles help hold the abdominal organs in place. If these muscles are not toned and strong, it is impossible to tilt your pelvis, which adversely affects your posture and alignment.

PELVIC STABILITY
The ability to keep the pelvis in neutral while moving your limbs.

POSTURAL ALIGNMENT
See Alignment

RIBCAGE BREATHING
A type of deep breathing that activates the muscles used to create core stability—the intercostal muscles, the deep muscles of the torso, and the pelvic floor muscles.

SACRUM
The posterior, wedge-shaped bone that forms part of the pelvis made from five fused vertebrae. If you place your hand on your spine, just above the buttocks, you can feel a slightly protruding bone, which is the sacrum.

SOFT
When a joint, such as the knee or elbow is extended but relaxed, it is soft.

TAILBONE
Also known as the coccyx, it is made up of three or four fused vertebrae at the base of the spine beneath the sacrum, located between the buttocks.

THORACIC
A term that relates to the 12 vertebrae of the upper back. These vertebrae connect with the 12 pairs of ribs that enclose and protect the chest cavity.

INDEX

continued on next page